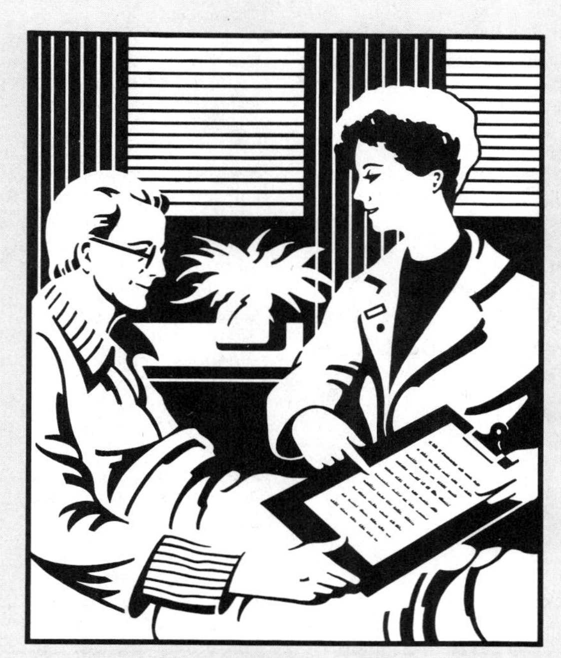

HOW TO TEACH PATIENTS

Springhouse Corporation
Springhouse, Pennsylvania

STAFF FOR THIS VOLUME

CLINICAL STAFF
Clinical Director
Barbara McVan, RN

Clinical Editors
Joanne Patzek DaCunha, RN, BS (project editor); Julie Tackenberg, RN, MA, CNRN

PUBLICATION STAFF
Executive Director, Editorial
Stanley E. Loeb

Executive Director, Creative Services
Jean Robinson

Editorial Director
Matthew Cahill

Editors
Catherine E. Harold (project editor), Peter Johnson

Copy Editors
David Prout (manager), Jane V. Cray

Design
John Hubbard (art director), Stephanie Peters (associate art director), Lorraine Carbo

Art Production
Robert Perry (manager), Anna Brindisi, Loretta Caruso, Don Knauss, Bob Wieder

Typography
David C. Kosten (manager), Diane Paluba (assistant manager), Joyce Rossi Biletz, Brenda Mayer, Robin Rantz, Brent Rinedoller, Valerie Rosenberger

Manufacturing
Deborah C. Meiris (manager), T.A. Landis

Production Coordination
Aline S. Miller (manager), Laurie J. Sander

The clinical procedures described and recommended in this publication are based on research and consultation with nursing, medical, and legal authorities. To the best of our knowledge, these procedures reflect currently accepted practice; nevertheless, they can't be considered absolute and universal recommendations. For individual application, all recommendations must be considered in light of the patient's clinical condition and, before administration of new or infrequently used drugs, in light of latest package-insert information. The authors and the publisher disclaim responsibility for any adverse effects resulting directly or indirectly from the suggested procedures, from any undetected errors, or from the reader's misunderstanding of the text.

Adapted from *Patient Teaching* (Nurse's Reference Library®), © 1987 by Springhouse Corporation.

ISBN 0-87434-170-1
HTP-011288

Library of Congress Cataloging-in-Publication Data
How to Teach Patients.
p. cm.
"Adapted from Patient teaching (Nurse's reference library), © 1987"—T.p. verso.
Bibliography: p.
Includes index.
1. Patient education—Study and teaching. I. Springhouse Corporation. II. Patient teaching.
[DNLM: 1. Patient Education—methods—nurses' instruction. W 85 H847]
RT90.H68 1989
615.5'07—dc19
DNLM/DLC
for Library of Congress 88-39680
ISBN 0-87434-170-1 CIP

CONTENTS

CONTRIBUTORS AND CLINICAL CONSULTANTS

At the time of publication, the contributors and clinical consultants held the following positions.

Contributors

Charmaine Cummings, RN, MSN
Clinical Nurse Educator
Neurology, Eye and Aging Research Nursing Service
National Institutes of Health
Bethesda, Md.

Gerri George, RN, MSN
President and Co-founder
SBI/Some Body Maternity Fitness Program
Bala Cynwyd, Pa.

Janice F. Hansen, RN, C, MA
Patient and Community Health Education Coordinator
Rutland Regional Medical Center
Rutland, Vt.

Pamela Rowe, RN, BSN, MEd
Assistant Director for Nursing Education
Mary Hitchcock Memorial Hospital
Hanover, N.H.

Ellen Shipes, RN, MN, ET(C), MEd
Clinical Nurse Specialist
Enterostomal Therapy
Vanderbilt University Hospital
Nashville, Tenn.

Joan E. Watson, RN, PhD
Assistant Professor
Graduate Program in Nursing Education
School of Nursing
University of Pittsburgh

Consultants

Ann R. Miller, RN, MS
Ambulatory Nurse Specialist
Beth Israel Hospital
Boston

Dorothy A. Ruzicki, RN, PhD
Patient Education/Research Coordinator
Sacred Heart Medical Center
Spokane, Wash.

Janice Selekman, RN, DNSc
Associate Professor
Thomas Jefferson University
Philadelphia

FOREWORD

More than ever before, your responsibilities are likely to involve patient teaching—especially in light of increasing professional, fiscal, and legal demands for improved patient education. But have your teaching skills kept pace with these growing demands? Do you feel confident in your role as a teacher? Are you sometimes uncertain about the best way to present information—or about the best way to evaluate whether your patient has truly learned?

Now, there's help at hand. *How to Teach Patients* offers clear advice and timesaving tips that will help you teach patients effectively and efficiently. That's especially important because effective teaching provides two major benefits for patients. It makes them more self-sufficient by bolstering their confidence in caring for themselves. What's more, it teaches them to anticipate complications and seek medical attention early—at times preventing rehospitalization.

How to Teach Patients begins with a chapter on basic principles of teaching and learning: how people learn best and differences in learning styles. It also discusses the legal implications of patient teaching.

After this introductory chapter, Chapters 2 to 4 parallel the nursing process. Chapter 2 covers patients' learning needs, providing directions for assessing both typical and problematic patients, including those of differing ages, levels of education, physical and mental abilities, and handicaps. Chapter 3 explains how to plan and effectively implement your teaching. It will also help you develop a workable teaching plan and show you the best ways to carry it out. The next chapter, on evaluation, explains how to gauge what the patient has learned and how well you've taught.

The following two chapters consider special topics. Chapter 5 covers the core information you'll have to teach each patient, such as an explanation of the disorder, preparation for diagnostic tests, or preoperative and postoperative care measures. Chapter 6 covers health promotion, with advice on diet, exercise, accident prevention, and other considerations for maintaining lifelong health.

Throughout the book, you'll find numerous charts, illustrations, and special features that will clarify important concepts and provide useful supplementary information. You'll also find home-care aids that can be copied and distributed to patients or their caregivers. In effect, the book provides you with all the tools you need to teach patients efficiently and effectively.

1 Understanding basic concepts

Introduction

In the past, we've taught patients because they've needed to know about their illnesses, their tests and treatments, and their home care regimens. Today, we still teach for the same reasons. But we do so with a new outlook on teaching brought about by growing professional, fiscal, and legislative demands for more efficient patient education. More than ever before, we need to be masterful teachers, learning and practicing the most effective techniques.

What is patient teaching?

First of all, it's something we do formally, with planning and deliberation. We also do it informally, whenever we take time to answer a patient's spontaneous question. We do it through explanation, demonstration, role playing, and teamwork.

Teaching, in effect, is an active process that aims to produce an observable change in the patient's behavior or attitude. The key words here are *active, process,* and *change.*

Active reflects the need for the patient's involvement. *Process* signals an ongoing series of actions or events that aim to help the patient learn how to maintain or improve his current health status. And *change* refers to acquiring new knowledge, new skills, or new values or beliefs.

How to teach effectively

To be effective teachers, we must do our own homework. We must control the learning environment, establish priorities for what our patients need to learn, supply instructional materials, and enlist the help of other staff members. We must also use appropriate teaching techniques and evaluate their outcome. More often than not, we do prepare for teaching, perhaps unconsciously. For example, by providing privacy while teaching, we control the learning environment and help reduce the patient's anxiety. By deciding that a newly diagnosed diabetic needs to learn injection technique and site rotation before leg and foot care, we establish priorities for learning. By supplying him with pictures and pamphlets, we reinforce or supplement our oral teaching.

Besides doing our homework, we need to look at our "classroom" to be effective teachers. A hospital or clinic, after all, isn't usually an inviting place for learning. Its staff, rules, and rituals are typically unfamiliar to the patient. As a result, the patient often feels especially vulnerable, creating a barrier to learning that we must overcome to teach effectively.

In contrast to the emotional distance a hospital or clinic setting invites, the relationship between ourselves and patients is likely to be closer than that between most teachers and learners. As nurses, we provide both physical and emotional care, allowing an intimacy rarely found in other teaching situations.

Who benefits from effective teaching?

The patient, of course. He benefits by learning how to maintain or improve his current condition. However, because the patient is the targeted beneficiary of this process, we typically evaluate teaching solely on the change produced in his attitude or behavior. Teaching, though, is a reciprocal activity: you may change your teaching methods as a result of the patient's feedback.

You and your patient aren't the only ones who benefit. Effective teaching also benefits the entire health care system. Research is beginning to show that the patient who has been taught about his condition and treatment seems to be leaving the hospital earlier. And the patient who's better able to understand and implement his home care plan has allowed more efficient use of personnel and equipment.

Thus, the hospital, clinic, and community as a whole can benefit from effective patient teaching.

THE CLIMATE FOR TEACHING

The changing direction of patient teaching

Within the past decade, various socioeconomic factors, role redefinitions, and revised professional standards have combined to change the direction of our teaching efforts. Perhaps the two areas of greatest change involve the patient's role as an active participant in health care and our role in assessing learning needs and planning to meet them.

The patient as participant

In the past, our teaching efforts usually focused on gaining the patient's passive compliance with the prescribed medical regimen.

Today, the thrust of our efforts has shifted toward promoting the patient's active involvement in his care plan.

What brought about this shift in emphasis? One factor is the growing consumer awareness of health care issues and services. For example, today's patient is more likely to seek a second opinion before surgery or to ask for explanations of drug effects. The mother of a child with chronic otitis media may tell the doctor, "Don't start Billy on that antibiotic—he's never responded to it in the past and we'll just waste time." Before, she probably would have automatically followed the doctor's orders rather than pose objections.

Of course, not all of your patients will be as assertive as Billy's mother. Rather, most patients you encounter will probably fall somewhere in the middle—between a passive learner and an active one. This middle group of patients, though, can be favorably influenced by teaching that's well planned and well carried out.

Patient's bill of rights

In 1972, the American Hospital Association gave formal support to this new participatory outlook by publishing "A Patient's Bill of Rights." While not a legal document, this bill attempts to set a standard for state-of-the-art health care and to ensure quality care and greater satisfaction for both patient and health care provider. Seven statements in the "Bill of Rights" deal with information the patient receives and accord him the right to know about his health problem, health status, treatments, alternative care measures, continuing care requirements, and hospital regulations. This recognition of the patient's right to information promotes his participation in his health care. It also challenges nurses to assess the patient's readiness to learn and to incorporate the patient's goals into the care plan.

Changes in the health care payment system

Another major influence on your teaching role has come from the legislative response to soaring health care costs. These escalating costs, especially Medicare costs, have resulted from a *retrospective* payment system—a system that paid for care after it was provided and failed to discourage inefficient use of personnel, time, and equipment. In 1983, the U.S. government's Health Care Financing Administration responded by developing a *prospective* payment system—a system that pays a fixed fee, established in advance, for a specific illness, or diagnosis-related group (DRG). This system has dramatically affected medical and nursing practice and has shortened the average hospital stay.

Under this new system, patients may be discharged from the hospital even though they require continued care at home, which, of course, increases the demand for timely and effective teaching. Patients may undergo batteries of diagnostic tests and procedures as outpatients, which naturally doesn't reduce, and in fact often increases, their teaching needs. Patients may also undergo same-day surgery, but they and their families now need to know about postoperative care measures imperative to safety and comfort—such as positioning after a tonsillectomy and administration of analgesics.

Shortened hospital stays require intensive patient teaching, as well as planning for follow-up care and teaching by someone other than the care planner, such as a home health nurse. Because of decreased time with the patient and his family in the hospital, we nurses need to teach "survival skills" first—those skills that the patient must have to care for himself safely and effectively upon discharge. As a result, we need to set priorities in our teaching plan.

Growing numbers of acutely ill patients

Under DRGs, the hospitalized patient today is usually more acutely ill than in the past. This means that his physiologic needs are necessarily more complex, which puts an even greater burden on your time. Understandably, you may find it difficult to monitor one patient with renal failure, provide wound care for another, balance fluids and electrolytes in a third, and still teach a fourth about respiratory distress syndrome. Setting priorities in situations like these isn't easy, but it's necessary.

Even given enough time and your commitment to teach, you may still be faced with a patient so ill that you question his ability and readiness to learn.

Increased longevity

Medical advances have helped significantly extend life expectancy and, as a result, have increased the number of chronically ill patients. And because many of these patients live independently and assume responsibility for their own care, they need to become willing partners in planning it. Our responsibility is increasingly to teach these patients self-care in a way that encourages collaboration and mutual problem solving. For example, in teaching an elderly diabetic about proper nutrition and exercise, you'll need to recognize the patient's preferences and test the feasibility of your instructions. In teaching a Parkinson's patient about safety, you'll need to know about his willingness and ability to modify his home environment to facilitate daily activities.

THE CHALLENGE OF TEACHING ACUTELY ILL PATIENTS

Because the typical hospitalized patient today is more acutely ill than in the past, you're facing a challenge in providing appropriate teaching. The patient's physical care alone can demand such large blocks of your time and can involve such complex equipment and procedures that teaching often is incomplete or, worse yet, not done at all.

The illustration here shows the range of demands acute illness places on the patient and you. These demands underscore the need for planning your teaching carefully to make learning effective.

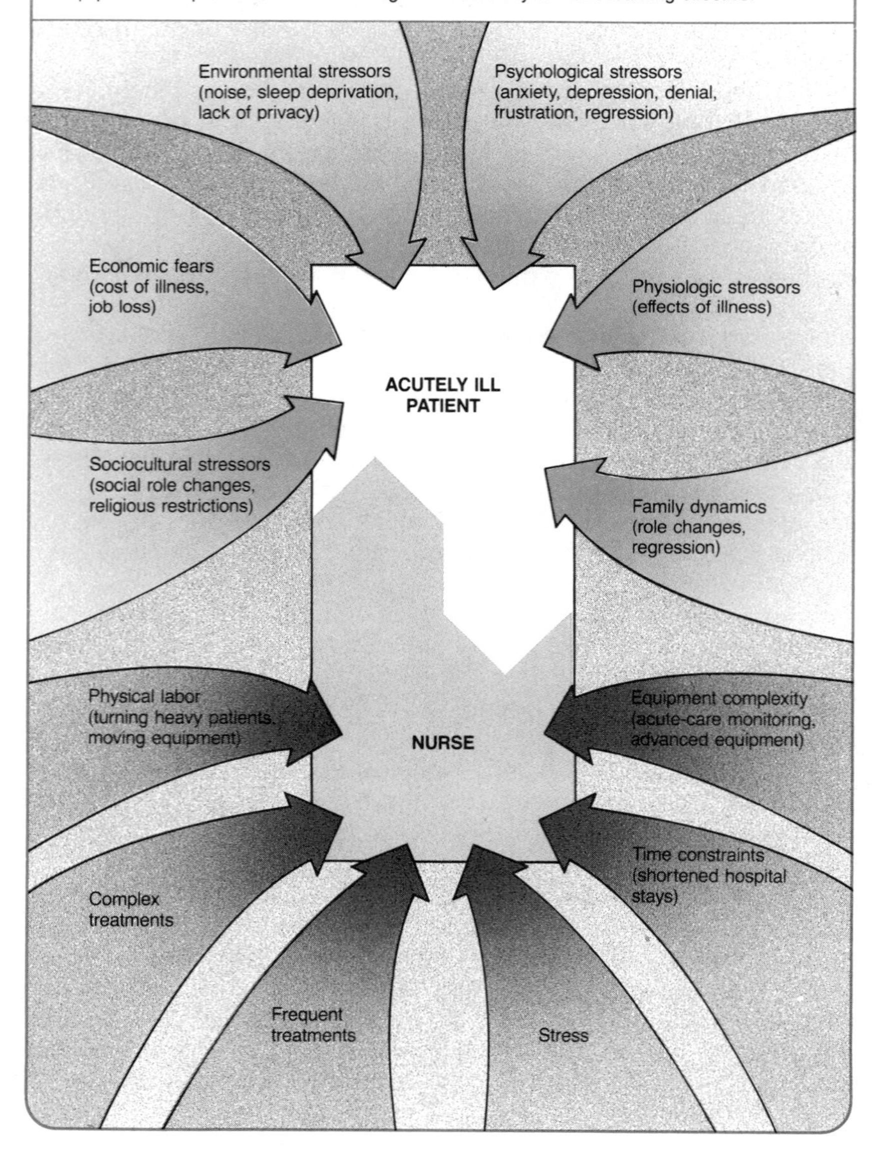

Legal implications for nurses

Greater patient participation in health care has led to an informed-consent philosophy, which promotes educated decision making by patients. In the past, for example, an epileptic patient was told when to take his medication; if he failed to take it as directed, he was considered noncompliant. Today, an epileptic patient can help plan medication regimens around his own life-style needs and identified trigger factors. Similarly, an epileptic patient who decides to stop her anticonvulsant medication while pregnant, if adequately informed, is no longer considered noncompliant but to be making a personal health decision.

In effect, we're now educating patients so they can make better decisions about their health care and assume greater responsibility for it. However, we still bear the responsibility for providing appropriate teaching.

Nurse practice act

The legal basis for our patient-teaching responsibilities rests in the nurse practice act. Although somewhat different from state to state, this act establishes licensing procedures and defines the practice of nursing within each state's jurisdiction. These guidelines for practice describe the nurse's participation in health education and are regarded as a professional standard.

Using the nurse practice act and the patient's bill of rights, the courts have placed responsibility on the nurse for timely and appropriate teaching. Several cases clearly illustrate this point. For example, in the 1944 case *Bernard v. Gravois,* a family alleged that a nurse failed to teach them how to use an electric heating pad correctly and that because of her oversight the patient burned himself. However, the court decided that the nurse had indeed given proper instruction and that the patient's injury occurred when a family member negligently carried out the instructions.

A Louisiana court ruled on a similar issue in 1983 *(Crawford v. Earl K. Long Hospital et al.).* The case involved a young boy who had been struck in the head with a baseball bat. The boy was examined by a doctor in the emergency department and found asymptomatic. The doctor then told a nurse to telephone the boy's mother and ask her to have someone take the boy home. The mother came to the hospital and took her son home. The next morning, she found him dead. In court, the mother alleged that she was given no instructions by the nurse or doctor to wake her son at regular intervals to check for arousability and coherence. But the nurse testified that she had indeed instructed the patient's mother. In fact, she pointed out that she had insisted for instructional purposes that the mother come to the hospital to pick up her son instead of letting the boy return home in a taxi, as the mother had requested.

In both of these cases, the court absolved the nurse of liability for the patient's poor outcome, with the verdict hinging on her implementation of teaching responsibilities.

A safeguard

Clear, complete documentation provides your legal protection if a patient claims he was harmed by improper teaching. In fact, failure to properly document your teaching can be interpreted in a court of law to suggest that you provided substandard nursing care even if you taught the patient thoroughly and felt confident about his response. So, complete documentation of your teaching and the patient's response to it represents your best defense against malpractice claims. An old saying can be applied to patient teaching: if you didn't document it, you didn't teach it.

TEACHING AND LEARNING

How nurses teach

Learning takes place through a planned sequence of activities. These activities can be formal—such as structured individual or group teaching sessions—or informal—such as conversations and the incidental instructions that are given during routine patient care. Whether carried out formally or informally, the teaching process goes through four steps familiar to every nurse: assessing, planning, implementing, and evaluating. But accomplishing these tasks involves more than just providing the patient with information.

Assessing

A careful assessment of your patient's learning ability and his learning needs related to his health problem forms the cornerstone of effective

HOW THE TEACHING PROCESS PARALLELS THE NURSING PROCESS

The steps of the teaching process parallel those of the nursing process, but they take a different slant. The nursing process emphasizes planning and implementing care based on assessing the patient's physical and psychosocial needs. The teaching process identifies teaching content and methods based on assessing the patient's learning needs. Both processes are circular, with ongoing assessment and evaluation constantly redirecting your planning and teaching.

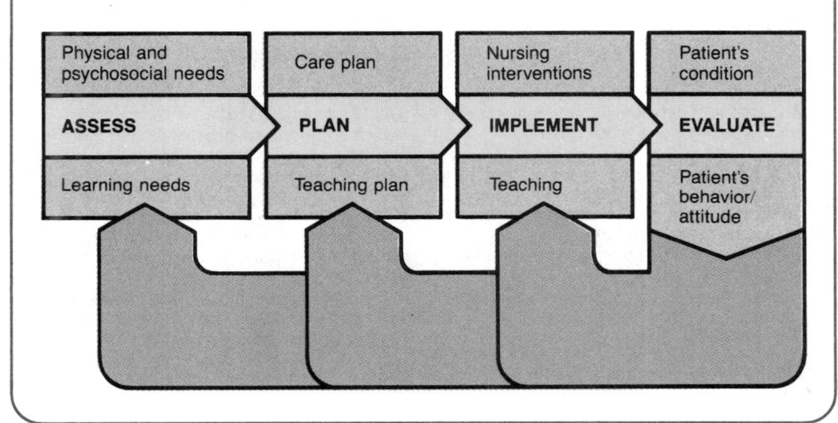

patient education and must precede any teaching. Your assessment must also address the patient's emotional readiness to learn. Trying to teach a patient about ostomy pouch application without recognizing that he's still unwilling to look at his stoma can only frustrate both you and the patient. This patient isn't emotionally prepared to learn the procedure even if it *is* on the teaching plan.

Assessment necessarily includes interviewing the patient's family members. This is most important when the patient is a young child or is mentally incapacitated, since you'll be directing most of your teaching to the family. In general, however, viewing the patient as a member of his family is vital to the teaching process, since the family network has the potential to facilitate or hinder your teaching efforts.

Assessing family dynamics—the way family members relate to the patient and to each other—will also help you tailor your teaching plan to the patient's learning needs. The wife who says, "Let me tell him what the tests show," or the husband who says, "I don't want my daughter to know her mother has cancer just yet," is regulating the flow of information among family members. Such regulation affects the way the patient and family adapt to a crisis.

Of course, the family is a dynamic unit. Its function and reliability as a unit will change as each member reacts to various stressors throughout the patient's hospitalization. Not all families have the ability to maintain cohesion and the growth of their members, and these families especially can present a formidable teaching problem. For example, attempting to teach a behavior modification program to the divorced parents of a head-injured child can be difficult if poor communication exists between the parents. Continuity of care

DOCUMENTING YOUR TEACHING

Accurate and detailed documentation helps ensure continuity in teaching. It tells other members of the health care team what has been planned for the patient, what has already been carried out, and what remains to be done. It ensures that no one duplicates teaching efforts.

Careful documentation also protects you legally. If the patient claims he was harmed because you supplied inadequate instructions or provided none at all, your legal protection rests on documentation of your teaching and the patient's response. Documentation can support your judgment in setting priorities for learner needs, selecting teaching methods, and evaluating learned tasks. For instance, statements of your patient's willingness and ability to learn can support your suggestion that certain teaching be done at a later date or even after discharge.

The following example—for a patient with Parkinson's disease—shows the kind of information you should document.

1. Patient's name and social security number on every record page
2. Date and time of each teaching session
3. Patient's health status and corresponding learning needs
4. Precise learning goal(s) agreed on by health care team and patient
5. Identified learning enhancements
6. Actual teaching you carry out
7. Specific teaching methods you use
8. Patient's characteristics as a learner
9. Precise description of exactly what occurred, avoiding broad terms such as "learned well" and "seems to understand"
10. Your evaluation of patient's change or learning
11. Patient's response to teaching/learning experience, using his own words and behaviors
12. Specific teaching materials you use
13. Indications that patient or family member understands instructions
14. Identified learning barriers
15. Final progress notes with discharge teaching about diet, medications, physical activity, and follow-up care
16. Legible writing
17. Your signature

may be affected when each parent interprets the program according to a personal perception of the child.

A family's learning readiness and needs require ongoing assessment. That's because the family's willingness and ability to learn will affect the patient's learning progress. So, when dealing with the patient's family, be sure to observe both verbal and nonverbal communication. Doing this will help you identify family members who

Westphal, Joseph [1]
SS 860-46-3954

Date [2] Time
1-14-89 0900

[3]
64 y.o. man c̄ newly diagnosed Parkinson's requiring flexibility exercises for mobility. Pt + health care team have agreed on exercise program. Pt has agreed to perform exercises b.i.d. to his level of tolerance. [4] Pt exhibits positive coping mechanisms + personal relations, which should aid learning.
[5] Maggi Breezler, RN

1100 [6] [7]
Flexibility exercises initiated c̄ explanation + demonstration of upper extremity activities. Explanation presented separately from questions, as pt prefers to "understand what to do ā doing the activity. [8] Pt return demonstrated [9] exercises under supervision + then independently s̄ error. [10] Pt states he knows how to do the exercises. Illustrated [12] examples left c̄ pt for his review. [11]
Maggi Breezler, RN

1500
Pt needs assistance c̄ transfer to chair. On-off syndrome being considered by M.D. Lower extremity exercises discussed + demonstrated. Pt unable to perform exercises. Pt correctly [13] indicates yes-no regarding execution of these exercises. Will evaluate actual performance of exercises at another time.
Maggi Breezler, RN

1-19-89
1400
Pt states, "Exercises are no use. This disease will stop me whenever it wants." Pt anger at disease presenting a barrier [14] to discharge teaching. Discharge planning + teaching being done c̄ wife until pt willing to participate. Discharge instructions given to wife, who demonstrates knowledge of information [15] by correctly responding to questions. Arrangements made c̄ community nurse for home safety evaluation. [16]
Maggi Breezler, RN
[17]

can hinder the patient's learning and thus require you to modify your teaching plan. It will also help you identify family members who can provide you with accurate information about the patient and can support him when you're implementing the teaching plan. Often a family member can persuade a patient to follow instructions or to attempt procedures he refused to try for you.

Planning

As a teacher, one of your roles is to design a plan that enhances patient learning. To do this effectively, you'll need to clarify objectives, set priorities, and organize information. In addition, you'll need to choose appropriate teaching methods and select supporting material.

Your teaching plan should include specific learning goals that you and your patient have agreed upon and the teaching strategies that will best help him meet these goals. For an ostomy patient, you're responsible for deciding which tasks he's ready to learn now and which need to be postponed until he's emotionally ready. For a same-day surgery patient, you're responsible for ensuring continuity of care by providing a mechanism for follow-up teaching.

Implementing

Actually carrying out your teaching plan necessarily involves all the other steps in the teaching process. As you interact with the patient, you're constantly reassessing how well he's learning and then planning again to make your teaching more effective.

Evaluating

The final step in the teaching process leads you to examine how well the patient has learned the necessary material—and, by extension, how well you've taught it. Often, evaluation restarts the teaching process, because it provides direction for changes in the other three steps that can help your patient meet his established learning goals. It also enables you to refine your skills as a teacher and to develop more effective methods.

Documenting

One goal of your teaching plan is to provide continuity of care for your patient. And one way to accomplish this is through careful documentation.

Your documentation should reveal what teaching you've planned and accomplished, and what the patient has learned. This information saves time and prevents duplication of patient-teaching activities. It allows other members of the health care team to begin instruction where you've left off—something that's especially important in units with floating staff and frequent reassignments.

• ***What to include.*** Since 1976, the Joint Commission on Accreditation of Healthcare Organizations (JCAHO) has mandated that medical records show evidence of informed consent and final progress notes. These notes should include specific instructions to the patient and/or his family about physical activity, medication, diet, and follow-up care.

The JCAHO requires documentation that the patient not only received instruction in these areas but also understood it. This documentation must include the patient's response to teaching and an assessment of his progress toward learning goals.

With this information, it's possible for you and others to evaluate teaching effectiveness. (See *Documenting Your Teaching,* pages 10 and 11.)

How your teaching approach affects learning

So much of the teaching process rests on accurate assessment of the patient's learning readiness and ability. Thus, understanding the developmental stages of personality can aid your assessment: you can assess the patient against models of psychosocial and intellectual (cognitive) development.

All aspects of development are continuous, concurrent, and interrelated. Just as a person follows a pattern of physical growth and development, he also follows patterns of emotional, psychological, and cognitive development. These patterns conform to stages, and the characteristics of growth (developmental tasks) within the stages have been described by Erikson, Piaget, and others. The patient's level of physical, emotional, and psychological development directly influences his readiness and willingness to learn.

Erikson's developmental stages

Psychoanalyst Erik Erikson describes the physical, emotional, and psychological stages of development and relates specific issues, or developmental work or *tasks,* to each stage. For example, if an infant's physical and emotional needs are met sufficiently, he completes his task—developing the ability to trust others. However, a person who's stymied in an attempt at task mastery may go on to the next stage but continue to carry with him the remnants of the unfinished task. For example, if a toddler isn't allowed to learn by doing, he develops a sense of shame and doubt in his abilities, which may complicate later attempts at independence. Similarly, a preschooler who's made to feel that the activities he initiates are bad may develop a sense of guilt that hinders his taking the initiative later in life. (See *Erikson's Stages of Development.*)

Piaget and cognition

Much of your teaching involves cognitive abilities: sharing information with the patient and looking for signs that he understands it. As a result, it's important to understand cognitive stages.

Child psychologist Jean Piaget describes the mechanism (cognition) by which the mind processes new information. Piaget says a person assimilates, or understands, whatever information fits into his established view of the world. When information doesn't fit, the person must reexamine and adjust his thinking to accommodate the new information. Piaget describes four stages of cognitive development and relates them to a person's ability to accommodate and assimilate new information.

The *sensorimotor* stage lasts from birth to 2 years. In it, the child learns about himself and his environment through motor and reflex actions. Thought derives from sensation and movement. The child learns that he's separate from his environment and that aspects of his environment—such as his parents or favorite toys—continue to exist even though they may be outside the reach of his senses. Your teaching, then, for a child in this stage should be geared to the sensorimotor system. You can modify behavior by using the senses: a frown, a stern or soothing voice—all serve as appropriate techniques to elicit desired behavior.

The *preoperational* stage begins about the time the child starts to talk and continues to about age 7. Using his new knowledge of language, the child begins to use symbols to represent objects, and early in this stage he also personifies objects. He's now better able to think about things and events that aren't immediately present. But he's unable to think through a series of actions; he still must perform them. Oriented to the present, the child has difficulty conceptualizing time. His thinking is influenced by fantasy—the way he'd like things to be—and he assumes that others see situations from his point of view. He assimilates information and then changes it in his mind to fit his ideas.

Because of the child's undeveloped sense of time and vivid fantasies, you'll be challenged to present information in a time frame that allows for questions and learning without fostering rumination.

ERIKSON'S STAGES OF DEVELOPMENT

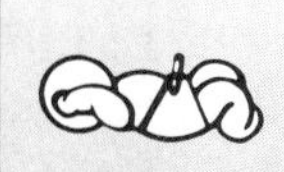

Infant
Trust vs. mistrust
Needs maximum comfort with minimal uncertainty in order to trust himself, others, and environment

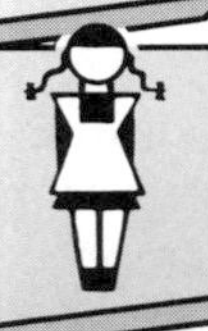

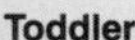

Toddler
Autonomy vs. shame and doubt
Works to master physical environment while maintaining self-esteem

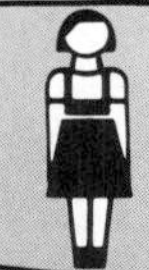

Preschooler
Initiative vs. guilt
Begins to initiate, not imitate, activities; develops conscience and sexual identity

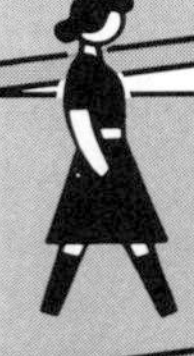

School-age child
Industry vs. inferiority
Tries to develop a sense of self-worth by refining skills

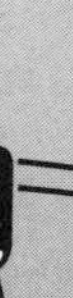

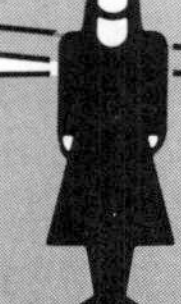

Adolescent
Identity vs. role confusion
Tries integrating many roles (child, sibling, student, athlete, worker) into a self-image under role model and peer pressure

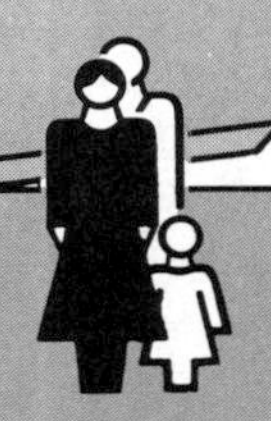

Young adult
Intimacy vs. isolation
Learns to make personal commitment to another as spouse, parent, partner

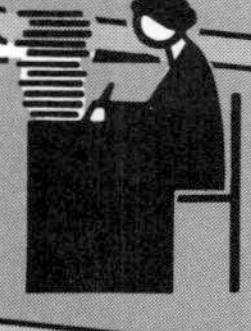

Middle-aged adult
Generativity vs. stagnation
Seeks satisfaction through productivity in career, family, civic interests

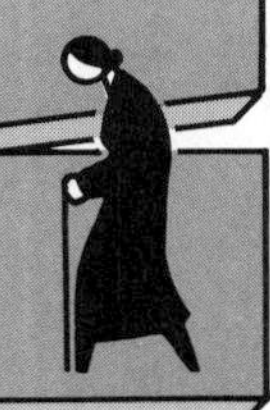

Older adult
Integrity vs. despair
Reviews life accomplishments, deals with loss and preparation for death

Using neutral words, body outlines, and equipment a child can touch gives him an active role in learning.

The *concrete* stage begins to appear at the time the child enters first grade and lasts into early adolescence. During this stage, accommodation increases. The child develops an ability to think abstractly and to make rational judgments about concrete or observable phenomena, which in the past he needed to physically manipulate to understand. Concrete objects must be within sight, however, for these thought processes to occur. In teaching this child, giving him the opportunity to ask questions and to explain things back to you allows him to mentally manipulate information.

The *formal operations* stage brings cognition to its final form during adolescence. A person reaches this stage when he no longer requires the physical presence of concrete objects to make rational judgments. At this point, he's capable of hypothetical and deductive reasoning. Teaching for the adolescent may be wide-ranging, since he'll be able to consider many perspectives.

Knowles and adult development

Using Piaget's and Erikson's work as a foundation, educator Malcolm Knowles has studied the adult learner. Not surprisingly, he feels that the adult learner has many of the cognitive abilities of Piaget's adolescent. However, Knowles considers an adult's life experiences as a crucial additional factor. He thinks that as the individual matures:

- his self-concept moves from dependency to self-direction.
- he accumulates a growing reservoir of experience that becomes a resource for learning.
- his readiness to learn becomes increasingly oriented to the developmental tasks of his various social roles.
- his time perspective changes from one of postponed application of knowledge to immediate application.
- his orientation to learning shifts from subject-centered to problem-centered.

If you examine personal and cognitive development and compare teaching approaches, you can see that children tend to be dependent as learners, while adults need to be independent and exercise control. For example, you'll usually teach an adult patient with migraine headaches some method of relaxation. Since an adult has more control over his time than a child does, you can logically allow him to decide which method fits his life-style and self-image. Of the possible methods, progressive muscle relaxation, which usually requires 10 to 20 minutes at a time to perform, may not appeal to a busy executive. Visualization may be more effective because it conforms to his time constraints.

Implications for assessment

Inaccurate assessment of a patient's developmental stage can misdirect your planning and hamper your teaching. For instance, not recognizing a 15-year-old's concern about his appearance and his standing among his peers may damage your rapport with him and create a learning barrier.

A complicating factor in your assessment is that chronologic age and developmental stage aren't always related. Throughout life, people move sequentially through developmental stages, but most also fluctuate somewhat among stages, often in response to outside stressors. These stressors, which include illness and hospitalization, can cause a person to temporarily regress to an earlier stage. Sometimes a person may not achieve the task expected of his chronologic age. So, you'll need to address your patient at his current developmental stage, not at the stage you'd expect him to be because of his chronologic age.

How to maximize your teaching effectiveness

In some situations, you'll have the time to sit down and develop a formal teaching plan. But in others, you'll be confronted with a "teachable moment" when the patient is ready to learn and is asking pointed questions. Invariably, these moments seem to come while you're in the midst of a dressing change or a catheterization. At times like these, you face a dilemma: to teach or not to teach. Having a knowledge of basic learning principles will help you take best advantage of these moments. Here are some principles proven to enhance teaching and learning.

Seize the moment

Teaching is most effective when it occurs in quick response to a need the learner feels. So, even though you're elbow deep in decubitus care, you should make every effort to teach the patient when he asks, "What can I do to stop getting so many open sores?" Your formal teaching plan may be in the patient's chart or in your desk and the slides may be in the head nurse's office, but the patient is ready to learn. So satisfy his immediate need for information now, and augment your teaching with more information later.

Involve the patient in goal setting

Merely presenting information to the patient doesn't ensure learning or change. For learning to occur, you'll need to get the patient actively involved in identifying his learning needs and goals. As the teaching process continues, you can further involve him by selecting

SAVING TIME FOR TEACHING

Sometimes, teaching patients what they need to know seems impractical—there's too much to cover and not enough time to do it. If you find yourself hard-pressed for time to teach, try using this method:

- List the patient's learning needs.
- Rank these needs: most important first, next most important second, and so on.
- Write your "teaching-to-be-done" list based on this ranking.

This method helps you distinguish the patient's *learning* needs from his *nursing care* needs. It also helps you organize your time and can quickly redirect your actions after an interruption.

Of course, the hardest part is ranking the patient's learning needs. To simplify this task, classify each learning need as:

- *immediate* (one that must be met promptly, such as teaching the patient who's being discharged in 2 hours) or *long range*
- *survival* (life-dependent, such as teaching the warning signs of adrenal crisis) or *related to well-being* (nice to know but not essential, such as describing the effects of stress in cardiovascular disease)
- *specific* (related to the patient's disorder or treatment, such as preparing him for upcoming cholecystectomy) or *general* (teaching that's done for every patient, such as explaining hospital visiting hours).

After you've classified the patient's learning needs, establish priorities. An immediate survival need, for example, would take top priority.

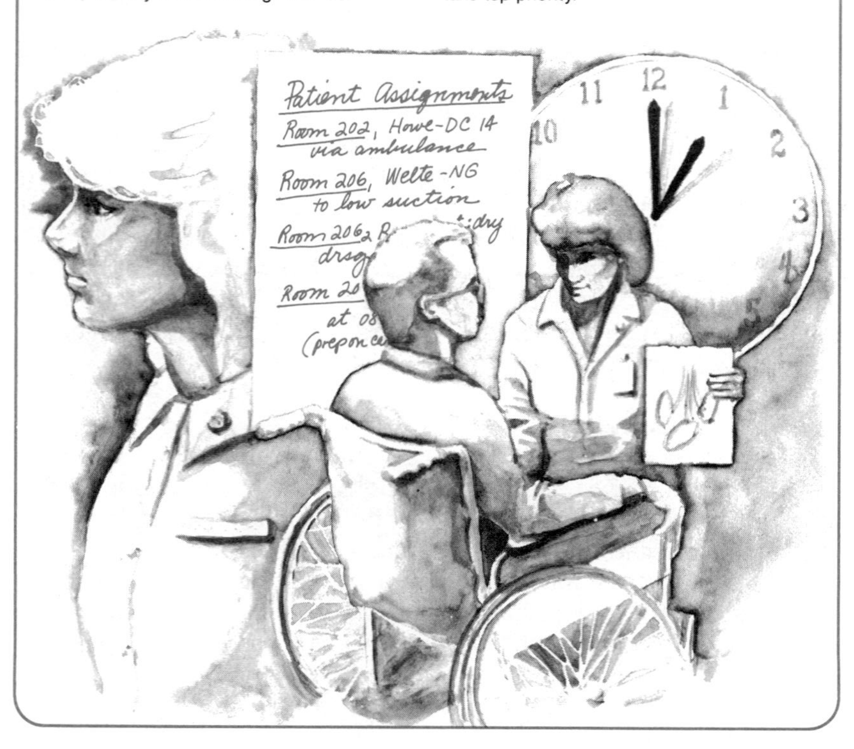

teaching strategies and materials that require his direct activity, such as role playing and return demonstration (see *Promoting Your Patient's Involvement in Learning,* page 20). Regardless of the teaching strategy used, giving the patient the chance to test his ideas, to take risks, and to be creative will promote learning.

Begin with what the patient knows

You'll find that learning moves faster when it builds on what the patient already knows. A patient who's been on peritoneal dialysis and now must undergo hemodialysis has some previous exposure to the concept of fluid exchange. Teaching that begins by comparing the old, known process and the new, unknown one will allow the patient to grasp new information quicker.

Move from simple to complex

The patient will also find learning more rewarding if he has the opportunity to master simple concepts first and then apply these concepts to more complex ones. Remember, however, that what one patient finds simple, another may find complex. A careful assessment will take these differences into account and help you plan the starting point for your teaching.

Accommodate the patient's preferred learning style

Learning styles and rates vary from one person to another. Besides being influenced by a person's intelligence and educational training, they're also influenced by preferences. *Visual* learners learn best by *seeing* or *reading* what you're trying to teach. *Auditory* learners learn best by *listening* to what you're teaching. *Tactile,* or *psychomotor,* learners learn best by *doing.*

You can improve your chances for teaching success if you assess your patient's preferred learning style, then plan teaching activities and use teaching tools appropriate to that style. To assess his learning style, you can observe him or simply ask him how he learns best. You can also experiment with different teaching tools, such as printed material, illustrations, videotapes, and actual equipment, to assess learning style. However, never assume that your patient can read well.

Sort goals by learning domain

You can combine your knowledge of the patient's preferred learning style with your knowledge of learning domains. (See *Understanding Learning Domains,* page 22.) Categorizing what he needs to learn into the proper domains helps identify and evaluate the behaviors you expect him to show.

PROMOTING YOUR PATIENT'S INVOLVEMENT IN LEARNING

Your patient will learn best when he's actively participating in the learning process. And he'll be most active when your teaching plan uses materials that simultaneously involve as many of his five senses as possible. You can review the illustration here to identify materials and the senses they involve.

SIGHT	SOUND	SMELL	TOUCH	TASTE
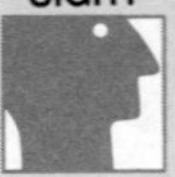	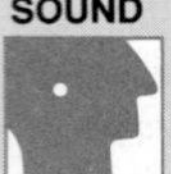	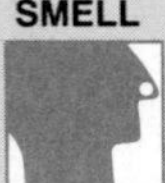	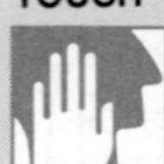	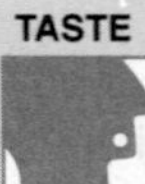
Written material Illustrations Slides	Lectures Audiotapes Records	Treatment solutions Oils Perfumes	Anatomic models Equipment	Food Spices

SIGHT AND SOUND

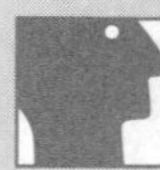
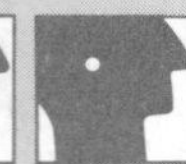

Role play
Videotapes
Television
Motion pictures

SIGHT, SOUND, AND TOUCH

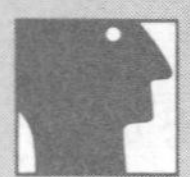
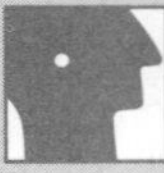
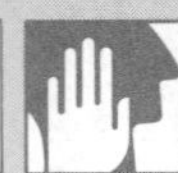

Working anatomic models

SIGHT, SOUND, TOUCH, AND SOMETIMES TASTE OR SMELL

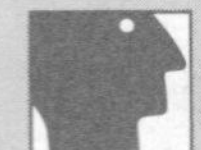
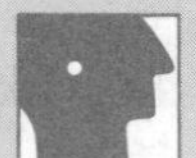
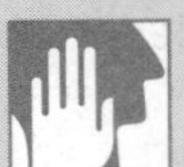
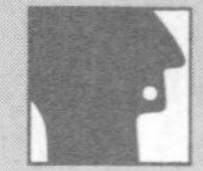
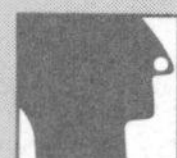

Demonstration
Return demonstration

ALL SENSES

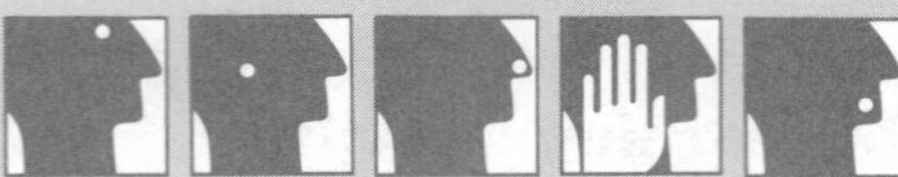

Repeated sensory learning experiences

Learning behaviors fall into three domains: cognitive, psychomotor, and affective. The *cognitive* domain deals with tasks that primarily reflect intellectual abilities. The *psychomotor* domain deals with tasks that are accomplished through physical or motor methods. The *affective* domain covers expression of feelings, attitudes, and values.

Most learning involves all three domains but isn't equally weighted. In teaching a patient about subcutaneous injection sites, recognize that the cognitive domain has the essential task: identifying the sites. The psychomotor and affective domains have less important tasks: finding the best site for a particular injection and expressing how the patient feels about this.

Make material meaningful

Another way to facilitate learning is to relate material to the patient's life-style—and to recognize incompatibilities. For example, teaching a hypertensive patient how to take his blood pressure may be futile if he perceives this as something his spouse ought to be doing. Similarly, discussing the need for a low-sodium diet with a traveling salesman may also be futile if he eats regularly in restaurants and feels unable to control the ingredients in his diet.

Allow immediate application of knowledge

Giving the patient the opportunity to promptly apply his new knowledge and skills reinforces learning and builds his confidence.

For instance, when you teach a mother how to perform postural drainage for her infant, you'll find that she'll learn better if she can quickly transfer what she's practiced on a doll to her own child (under your supervision, of course). This immediate application lets her translate her learning to the "real world" and provides an opportunity for problem solving, feedback, and emotional support.

Another example: providing sample menus to the diabetic patient helps reinforce his cognitive skills of food selection. This type of rehearsal reinforces his ability to select foods correctly on his own.

Plan for periodic rests

While you may want the patient to push ahead until he's learned everything on your teaching plan, remember that periodic plateaus occur normally in learning. When your instructions are especially complex or lengthy, your patient may feel overloaded and appear unreceptive to your teaching. Be sure to recognize these signs of mental fatigue and let the patient relax. (You, too, can use these periods—to review your teaching plan and make any necessary adjustments.)

UNDERSTANDING LEARNING DOMAINS

During the teaching process, you'll be carefully identifying what you want the patient to learn and evaluating if he's actually learned it. Understanding the learning domains can ease both steps.

Every task you want the patient to learn, such as ostomy care (shown in italics in the example here), falls primarily into one of three learning domains—cognitive, psychomotor, or affective. And within each domain, a task can be accomplished or learned on any of several progressively complex levels. Understanding the degree of ability and comprehension each level demands can help you identify the steps you'll have to take in guiding your patient toward his learning goals.

Understanding this, you'll find it easier to clarify learning goals, plan teaching strategies, and focus your evaluation.

COGNITIVE DOMAIN

Knowledge: Recalling information. *(Patient can list equipment needed for pouch change.)*

Comprehension: Understanding. *(Patient can state relation between ostomy care and skin integrity.)*

Application: Applying old information to new situations. *(Patient can recognize skin breakdown by recalling signs of past infection.)*

Analysis: Breaking down whole into parts. *(Patient can pinpoint problem, such as pouch leak.)*

Synthesis: Putting parts together to create a new whole. *(Patient can identify a solution, such as applying more pouch adhesive.)*

Evaluation: Judging the value of material for a given purpose. *(Patient can rate effectiveness of his solution to problem.)*

PSYCHOMOTOR DOMAIN

Perception: Becoming aware of a stimulus through the senses. *(Patient knows what equipment is needed for pouch change.)*

Set: Readiness for a particular physical action. *(Patient can handle equipment and ask questions.)*

Guided response: Performing overt behavior under supervision. *(Patient can follow pouch application instructions.)*

Mechanism: Learning a behavior to the point of habit. *(Patient can apply pouch correctly without instructions.)*

Complex overt response: Performing a complex motor pattern. *(Patient can incorporate local skin care into pouch application.)*

Adaptation: Altering a learned motor response to meet new problems. *(Patient can use same principles to apply different type of pouch.)*

Origination: Creating new motor patterns. *(Patient can cut pouch to fit.)*

AFFECTIVE DOMAIN

Receiving: Attending to and allowing continuation of a stimulus. *(Patient can look at stoma.)*

Responding: Responding voluntarily to a stimulus. *(Patient can ask and answer questions about stoma and pouch application.)*

Valuing: Accepting the value of a behavior to the point of acting it out. *(Patient's willing to perform pouch application.)*

Organization: Organizing behavioral framework based on values. *(Patient's willing to make time for stoma care.)*

Characterization: Expressing feelings that portray view of life. *(Patient shows self-esteem despite altered body image.)*

Tell the patient how he's progressing

Learning's made easier when you make the patient aware of his progress. This feedback can often motivate him to greater effort because it makes his goal seem attainable.

Also remember to ask your patient how he feels he's doing. He probably wants to take part in assessing his own progress toward learning goals. And his input can guide your feedback, since his reactions are often based on what "feels right."

Reward desired learning with praise

Praising desired behavior improves the chances of the patient's repeating that behavior. For example, a child with cystic fibrosis may have difficulty learning how to perform breathing exercises. But praising his success associates the desired learning goal with a feeling of growing competence in an appreciative atmosphere. It can reassure him that he's learned the technique, can help him refine it, and can motivate him to practice.

A FINAL WORD

For your teaching to be effective, the learning process must be dynamic, with your patient involved every step of the way. The extent of his involvement will depend greatly on how well you've identified his learning needs. And this, in turn, will depend on how completely and accurately you've assessed his developmental level, his ability to learn, and his receptivity to your teaching.

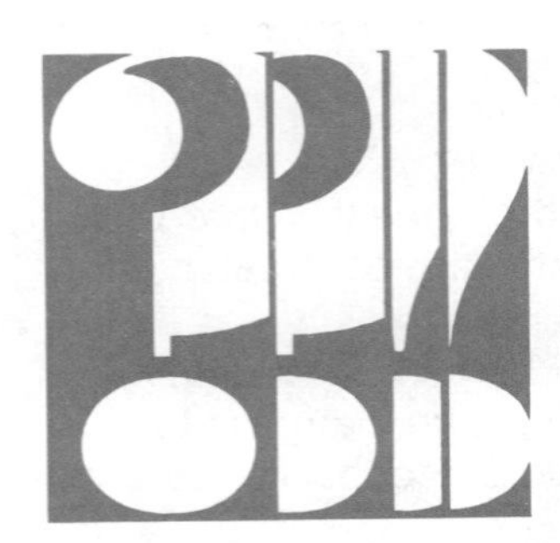

2

Assessing learning needs

Introduction

Like most nurses who've conscientiously tried to teach patients, you've probably been disappointed with the results at one time or another. Maybe you've felt that your message just wasn't getting through—for example, when a patient didn't follow your explicit instructions for taking his medication. Or perhaps you've felt that your teaching somehow missed its mark—for example, when you tried to teach a patient how to change a dressing but found that he just couldn't do it.

Assess before you teach

Often, you can avoid frustrations like these by carefully assessing your patient before you begin teaching. By assessing first, you can determine what your patient wants and needs to know. And you can determine what he's ready, willing, and able to learn. Knowing this information can make your teaching faster, easier, and more effective.

Careful assessment *saves you valuable teaching time.* It helps you pinpoint a patient's specific learning needs and evaluate his receptivity to learning, so you'll know what—and when—to teach. It also helps you establish your patient's learning priorities, so you'll know where to devote most of your teaching time.

Careful assessment *facilitates your teaching.* It allows you to discover possible barriers—physical, emotional, behavioral, or environmental—that may interfere with your teaching and inhibit learning. With this information, you can decide which teaching methods and tools are best to include in your teaching plan. Then you can modify your teaching techniques to meet your patient's individual needs.

Finally, careful assessment *makes your teaching more effective.* Once you've identified your patient's needs, you can tailor your teaching plan to make learning more meaningful to him. The result? He'll learn faster, retain the information longer, and be more likely to follow directions or change his behavior accordingly.

How to proceed

Your preteaching assessment begins with collecting information about the patient. Then, you'll need to assess the various factors that influence his readiness to learn—for example, his emotional state and personal learning goals. Next, you'll need to assess his willingness to learn and the factors that may affect it—for example, his health and religious beliefs. You'll also need to assess his ability to learn by identifying any factors that may enhance or impede learning—for example, his physical condition, intellectual abilities, and learning style.

THE TECHNIQUES

Collecting assessment data

Your preteaching assessment is an ongoing process—it won't be completed in one session. Each time you talk to a patient, check his chart, or attend a meeting with other members of his health care team, you gather information that can help you assess the patient's learning needs and abilities. When collecting assessment data, consider the following sources of information:
- interviews with the patient and his family
- written records, such as the patient's medical chart
- meetings with members of the health care team.

Interviewing the patient

You'll gather most of the information you need to complete a preteaching assessment during formal and informal interviews with the patient. *Formal interviews,* such as the health history you take when the patient's admitted to the hospital, provide a structured format for obtaining data. *Informal interviews* are the conversational exchanges that usually occur while you're providing routine care—for example, when you ask a postoperative patient how he's feeling while you change his dressing. Because they're less structured, informal interviews tend to be less threatening to the patient and often elicit his true thoughts and feelings. During both formal and informal interviews, remember to ask about the patient's past health experiences, current illness, and health expectations.
- ***Ask about the patient's past health experiences—both positive and negative.*** Is it unusual for the patient to be ill, or is he often bothered by health problems? When he's ill, does he like others to care for him, or does he prefer to care for himself? The patient's answers to these questions may reveal his customary reaction to illness—information that can help you choose the best approach for planning care and teaching. What's more, asking the patient about

FOUR STEPS TO TAKE BEFORE TEACHING

Before you begin teaching, you'll need to take four important steps. Your first step entails setting standards for what a patient should learn. And your last step entails formulating a statement of the patient's readiness, willingness, and ability to meet those standards—in effect, your teaching diagnosis. Between these steps, you'll collect and evaluate information. You'll probably also discover additional areas for teaching, based on what your patient and his family want to learn about his condition. If so, you'll need to reassess the patient or modify your teaching standard to create the best possible teaching plan.

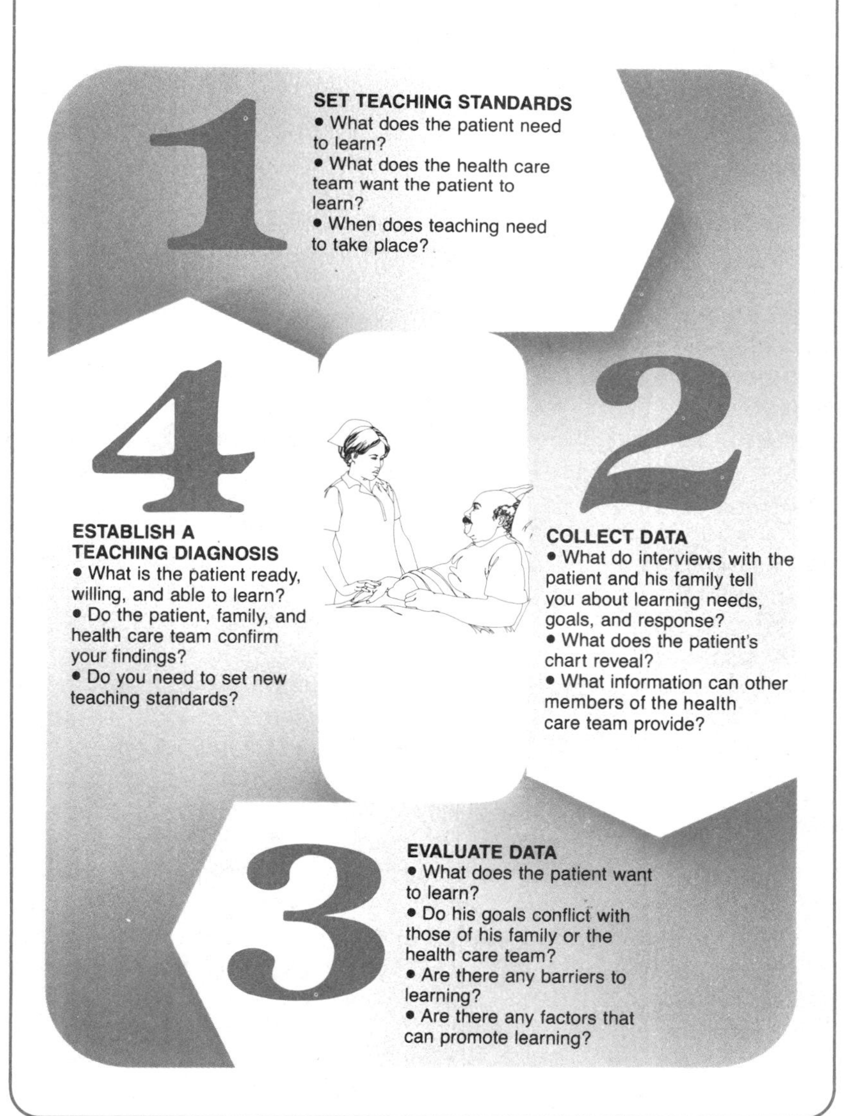

his past health experiences helps you assess his compliance with past care instructions.

• ***Ask about the patient's current illness.*** How much does the patient already know about his illness and its symptoms, and what additional information would he like to learn? By knowing the patient's perceived need for further learning, you can decide what to include in the teaching plan.

• ***Ask about the patient's health expectations.*** Try to find out how the patient thinks his present illness will affect his future health. This information helps you determine how well the patient has adjusted to his diagnosis and prognosis. It may also provide clues about the condition's impact on the patient and his family, and help point out the need for additional teaching and support measures.

Interviewing the patient's family

During your preteaching assessment, be sure to interview the patient's family or any close friends or companions who'll be involved in your teaching plan. The patient's family and close acquaintances not only help you validate and clarify the patient's history but also may point out a need for additional teaching—especially if they'll be involved in caring for the patient after he leaves the hospital.

• ***Assess the family's reaction.*** Try to determine how well the patient's family is coping with his hospitalization. Their reaction may color his response to learning. For example, suppose your patient's family is eager for him to "hurry up and get well," so he can return home and resume his customary role and responsibilities. Their eagerness may pressure the patient to tackle learning tasks before his condition permits. This could prolong the teaching process and spell frustration for both the patient and his family.

When the family understands the reason for a patient's treatment, they're more likely to support him as he acquires new information and skills. Generally, a patient's most likely to learn effectively when his family supports his efforts and shares a positive, realistic attitude.

When you interview the family, you'll also need to assess their understanding of the patient's diagnosis and prognosis. Are they well-informed, or do they have misconceptions that could interfere with your teaching? Have they accepted the diagnosis or are they unable to face it? Find out their goals for the patient's recovery and their perception of the patient's ability to learn. Are their expectations geared toward the patient's true capabilities?

Also ask the family about the patient's usual coping mechanisms. Often, they can provide insights into the patient's daily activities and coping mechanisms that the patient himself may overlook. Finally, assess the family's willingness to learn and participate in the patient's care. Do they ask pertinent questions about the patient's illness and need for care, or do they "tune out" during your explanations?

• ***Identify emotional needs.*** Sometimes you'll need to identify—and try to meet—some specific emotional need before you can effectively teach the patient's family. For example, if a patient's wife seems *hostile* during the interview, you may realize it's because she feels she's in the way—or because members of the health care team have pushed her away. These feelings are especially likely to surface if the patient needed her care at home, before his hospitalization. Once you've identified the wife's need to play a larger role in her husband's care, you can try to meet it while you teach—for example, by asking her to perform basic care techniques while you're explaining them.

Guilt can also interfere with the family's understanding of the patient's illness—especially if they think something they did or didn't do was responsible for the hospitalization. You can sometimes recognize this emotion by a family member's inattentiveness and questions. For example, suppose you're interviewing a woman whose elderly mother fell and struck her head, causing formation of a cerebrovascular clot, which required surgery. During the interview, you realize that the daughter clearly isn't paying attention. When you ask if there's anything else she'd like to know about her mother's condition, she asks several seemingly unimportant questions and then asks the "big" one: could she have kept the clot from forming if she'd put an ice bag on her mother's head? In cases like this, you'll need to relieve a family member's guilt before she'll be ready to learn what you need to teach her.

Conducting a successful interview

Successful interviewing involves listening, posing questions, and choosing words with care. It also requires you to assess nonverbal cues and to recognize how your attitudes and the environment affect the interviewing process.

• ***Be a good listener.*** The way you talk and listen to your patient and his family can enhance communication—or hinder it. For example, if you frequently interrupt the patient, you force him to reinitiate the conversation. The result? Not only will the patient feel you aren't listening but the message you receive will be disjointed.

• ***Pose questions carefully.*** By posing your questions carefully, you can encourage the patient and his family to continue talking, so you can learn as much as possible. You can also direct their responses to provide the type of information you need.

Asking an *open-ended question* generally garners the most information, since this type of question allows many possible answers. It also allows a person to clarify his thoughts and feelings or elaborate on them. For example, suppose a patient tells you that he hasn't felt comfortable since beginning a new treatment schedule. By responding with an open-ended question—such as "What is it about your schedule that makes you uncomfortable?"—you allow the patient to expound on his original statement. His response may also provide clues about his approach to problem solving, since open-ended questions often require a person to form a judgment.

In contrast, by responding with a *closed question*—such as "When did you begin your new treatment?"—you direct the patient toward providing specific information. Unlike an open-ended question, a closed question can usually be answered in just one or two ways. This type of question may require the patient simply to recall information or also to translate, interpret, and rephrase that information. His response may help you determine how well he remembers and understands what he's been taught.

• ***Watch your language.*** During the interview, keep in mind that your choice of words may keep you from getting the information you need. For example, using unfamiliar medical terms or jargon—such as *enuresis, stat,* and *NPO*—when readily understandable lay expressions exist can confuse the patient. Similarly, using familiar terms that have a double meaning, such as *dirty* and *sterile,* can also confuse him. However, if you must use a special term, such as *EKG* or *catheter,* be sure to explain it—or at least ask the person if he knows what it means. Remember, however, some people may be reluctant to admit they don't understand.

Using vague language can also hinder communication, create confusion, and sometimes result in an incorrect assessment. For example, suppose you're interviewing a patient who's receiving anticoagulant therapy. If you ask him whether he has experienced any "excessive or prolonged bleeding," he may say "no" simply because he doesn't understand how much bleeding is "excessive" or how long the bleeding must persist to be considered "prolonged."

• ***Watch the patient's language, too.*** By listening carefully to your patient's choice of words, you can adjust your vocabulary to his level of understanding. For example, if a patient says "pee" and you insist on using the word "urinate" or "void," the patient may not grasp your meaning. Having to constantly explain yourself will make both of you feel foolish. On the other hand, you may be led to believe a patient or family member who uses specialized medical terms is knowledgeable when he really isn't. In both situations, you must determine the person's level of understanding so you can communicate clearly with him.

KNOW YOURSELF: ASSESSMENT'S FIRST COMMANDMENT

Like most nurses, you probably find that teaching certain patients—or certain topics—makes you feel anxious or uneasy. Why? Possibly because they challenge your self-confidence as a nurse. Or perhaps because they trigger an emotional response based on your values or biases.

Your life experiences help shape your values, opinions, and expectations. But as a nurse, you can't allow them to interfere with the objective preteaching assessment each patient deserves. Do you, for example, disapprove of certain kinds of people, such as alcoholics or drug abusers? If so, you may unconsciously make careful assessment a lower priority for them than you would for other patients. Or you may omit certain assessment information or interpret it to match your preconceptions.

Do you dislike teaching certain procedures, such as stoma care? If so, your negative attitude may surface when you assess a patient who needs this teaching.

Do you find yourself agreeing with sweeping statements about:

- ethnic background, such as "The Irish are so stubborn; you can't teach them anything."
- sex, such as "Men don't need to talk about their problems the way women do."
- aging, such as "Old people can't learn new things or care for themselves."
- physical appearance, such as "If he weren't so fat, he'd have learned to walk with a cane by now."
- the effect of an unfavorable prognosis, such as "He has AIDS, so what's the point in teaching him about maintaining good nutrition?"

To keep biases like these from coloring your assessment, think about patients or teaching topics that have been challenging for you. What kind of person do you most dislike finding in your patient assignments? Which procedures are you uncomfortable teaching? Why do you think you feel this way?

Of course, you can't change the way you feel overnight. But you can learn to put your feelings into perspective and try to prevent them from compromising the way you assess—and teach—your patients.

Sometimes, you may have difficulty understanding what your patient or his family says—especially if they use slang or "street talk." This can keep you from developing a trusting relationship and completing your preteaching assessment. If a patient or a family member uses unfamiliar words, ask him to explain them. Or ask an appropriate colleague to help you communicate with the patient. (Some hospitals provide staff with special vocabulary lists that translate local slang into common language.)

- ***Assess nonverbal cues.*** Pay attention to the nonverbal cues—such as behavior, facial expressions, and gestures—that a patient sends during an interview. Sometimes, the nonverbal message a patient conveys may conflict with his verbal message. For example, a blank look may mean he hasn't understood what you've told him, even if he says he has.

Similarly, a patient's nonverbal actions can give very different meanings to the same words. For example, a patient who meets your eyes with a steady, determined look and says, "I'm just not getting any better," may be telling you that he's ready to learn about new treatment options. Another patient who says these same words but shrugs his shoulders, looks away, and begins to weep is communicating a very different message. He may be telling you that he thinks his situation is hopeless and that nothing you teach him will make a difference.

A patient's nonverbal cues can also indicate when a particular topic needs to be addressed in more detail—or when it needs to be shelved temporarily. For example, when you raise a sexually related topic, does the patient avoid eye contact or develop nervous mannerisms? If so, he's telling you with his actions that the topic is sensitive. By being aware of both verbal and nonverbal responses, you can determine if you need to probe further, change the subject, or stop asking questions.

• ***Be aware of your attitude.*** Your own feelings and values may influence not only the information you collect during the interview but also your interpretation of the patient's learning needs. Like everyone else, your feelings and values have been shaped by your past experiences. But as a nurse, you can't allow any biases to interfere with the objective assessment each patient deserves. Being aware of your own biases can help you recognize, anticipate, and avoid problems. During the interview, try to look at how your personal response to the patient is influencing the interviewing process. If it seems to be influencing it negatively, check your assessment findings with other members of the health care team. (See *Know Yourself: Assessment's First Commandment,* page 31.)

• ***Be aware of the hospital environment.*** Keep in mind that the hospital environment can also affect the accuracy of your preteaching assessment. For example, a room that's crowded or noisy is distracting and may prevent you and the patient or his family from concentrating. One that's too cold, too hot, or poorly lit also impedes assessment by causing discomfort. Lack of privacy may make the patient or his family reluctant to reveal personal or intimate details.

You may not always be able to create the ideal setting for an interview—an environment that's quiet, comfortable, and private. But do make an effort, especially to reduce distractions and to provide privacy. For example, if the patient's in a semiprivate room but ambulatory, take him to a quiet area outside the room. If he isn't ambulatory, draw the curtains around the bed and speak in a low tone to convey respect for his privacy. Or conduct the interview when his roommate's gone.

Reviewing written records

The patient's medical chart provides the data base for your preteaching assessment. His health history reveals his general physical and emotional state and educational level—factors that can greatly affect his readiness, willingness, and ability to learn. The patient's chart also outlines basic information about his diet, living situation, support systems, and usual daily activities—details that can affect his health practices after he leaves the hospital. Social service records and consultation sheets may also provide information about any family difficulties, emotional problems, or use of support services that can influence the patient's approach to learning. By regularly checking laboratory and radiology reports, nurses' change-of-shift notes, and progress reports, you can continually update your assessment.

Meeting with the health care team

Formal and informal interviews with the patient's doctor and other health care team members expand and validate your preteaching assessment. Find out what your colleagues have learned from their interviews with the patient and his family. Do their impressions support or contradict your findings? Also find out what other health care team members have told the patient and his family about the patient's diagnosis, prognosis, and treatment plan. By clarifying these facts, you can avoid dispensing conflicting information to the patient and his family.

You can further enhance your preteaching assessment by attending regular multidisciplinary conferences with other members of the patient's health care team—his dietitian, physical therapist, or social worker, for example. If possible, also include the patient and his family in these meetings. Group conferences allow the health care team to share information about the patient and to set goals for his recovery or rehabilitation. They also provide a forum for resolving conflicts about teaching priorities.

THE LEARNER

Assessing readiness to learn

Various factors influence a patient's readiness to learn. During your assessment, consider the patient's current *emotional state,* his *stage of adaptation to his illness,* his *emotional maturity,* his *past life experiences,* and the *goals* he and his family want to reach. Assessing a patient's readiness to learn involves answering these questions:

• What information, if any, is the patient emotionally ready to learn at this time?
• How well has the patient adapted to his illness?
• Is the patient emotionally mature enough to take responsibility for learning?
• Have the patient's experiences helped prepare him to learn the concept or skill you're planning to teach?
• Do the patient and his family have realistic learning goals?

Most patients show that they're ready to learn by asking questions or by participating in care. If possible, plan to time your teaching to take advantage of your patient's readiness to learn. Not only will learning be more effective but your teaching task will be easier.

Emotional state

During your assessment, find out if the patient has any pressing emotional needs or any emotional problems that will require you to adapt your teaching techniques. A patient's emotional state affects not only the way he looks at the world but also his readiness to learn. For example, an overwhelming health problem can crush a patient's confidence in his ability to control his life, leaving him *depressed* about his illness and *apathetic* about learning. If he can't do anything about his illness, he feels, why should he bother learning about it? Another patient who feels *happy* about his progress and *hopeful* about his recovery will more likely be ready to learn how to achieve his goals.

A patient typically feels a variety of emotions that can affect his readiness to learn. Often, mild emotional responses speed learning. *Mild anxiety,* for example, occurs normally during learning and can sharpen a patient's attention, increasing his readiness to learn and understand. More intense emotional responses can overwhelm him and make him less receptive to teaching. Here are some common emotions hospitalized patients feel:

• ***Anxiety.*** A patient who feels threatened by his illness often reacts with anxiety. As his anxiety worsens, his perception of what's going on around him narrows; his goals become oriented toward gaining immediate relief rather than toward learning.

Often, a hospitalized patient's family experiences severe anxiety that can increase the patient's stress and create a barrier to learning. For example, suppose you're assessing the learning needs of a couple whose 5-year-old daughter has been admitted for possible leukemia. Naturally, their anxiety level is high. The father is impatient and abrupt when he speaks; he paces up and down and often becomes hostile during the interview. The mother acts nervous and edgy; she appears to have been crying and is on the verge of tears

RECOGNIZING COPING MECHANISMS

A patient may use coping mechanisms to protect himself from anxiety by changing, concealing, or falsifying the threat he believes a stressful event or condition poses. As you know, coping mechanisms aren't always harmful. But because they can interfere with a patient's learning, you need to recognize and understand them. This chart defines and describes some of the coping mechanisms patients commonly use.

COPING MECHANISM	DEFINITION	BEHAVIOR TRAITS	REASONS FOR USE
Denial	Refusing to recognize some aspect of reality	Denies known facts or reality of illness; refuses responsibility for learning self-care	Protects patient from painful reality
Rationalization	Justifying behavior by using a plausible excuse	Intensely defends own position	Maintains patient's self-respect and wards off guilt feelings
Displacement	Redirecting an emotion or impulse to another person or object	Focuses on teaching inconsistencies of health care team	Allows patient to express repressed feelings
Conversion	Translating psychological problems into physical complaints	Claims physical problems that have no clinical cause; requests self-care information related to physical problems	Helps patient avoid anxiety-producing situation because he's "ill"; gives patient legitimate reason for seeking help and support or removes focus from psychological problems
Regression	Returning to a previous, immature way of behaving	Refuses to participate in learning; performs previously learned tasks at a lower level of ability	Permits patient to avoid anxiety of real situation
Projection	Transferring unwanted thoughts and tendencies to others	Minimizes own guilt by making others feel guilty; blames others for own problems; makes others responsible for learning tasks or for own failure to learn	Provides an outlet for patient's repressed thoughts and tendencies

frequently during the interview. The daughter sits on her mother's lap throughout the interview, stroking her mother's arm and staring at her father. She seems bewildered and frightened. At this time, neither parent is ready to learn about their daughter's suspected illness. What's more, their anxiety heightens their daughter's stress, decreasing her readiness to learn on her own.

Some people try to protect themselves from anxiety through various coping mechanisms, such as denial or regression. You'll need to recognize when your patient's using coping mechanisms—they can make him less receptive to learning. (See *Recognizing Coping Mechanisms,* page 35.)

- ***Anger.*** A patient commonly becomes angry when he has unrealistic expectations of medical care. For example, he may express anger if he believes that he's not receiving sufficient care or not recovering quickly enough.
- ***Fear.*** A hospitalized patient may be prone to a variety of fears.

ASSESSING YOUR PATIENT'S STAGE OF ADAPTATION

When you interview your patient, try to determine how he feels about his illness. Does he deny its existence? Does he blame it on himself or others? Does he seem willing to accept it and modify his life-style?

Your patient may be experiencing any of these feelings about his illness. In fact, he may experience all of them, but at different times. By recognizing his response—or stage of adaptation—to his illness, you can avoid teaching him something he's not ready to learn. For example, if he's still in the initial stage of disbelief, you'll need to postpone teaching until he's ready to face the existence of his illness. This chart will help you recognize the six stages of adaptation patients commonly experience.

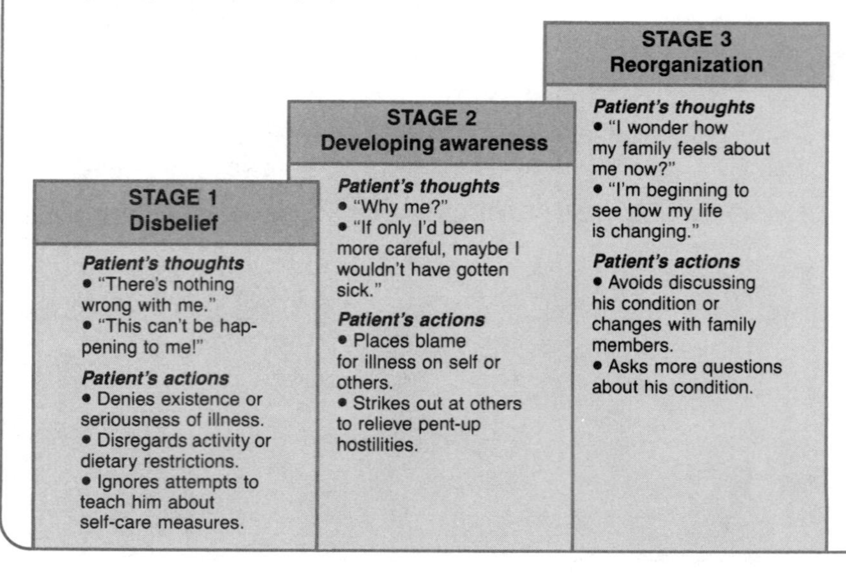

For example, a patient who's especially dependent on his family or friends may fear *loneliness.* Another patient may fear *financial instability* if his illness forces a realignment of family roles—such as when the homemaker must seek employment to support the family. And a patient who hasn't been fully informed about (or doesn't fully understand) his illness or treatment regimen may fear *the unknown.*

Sometimes, fear prevents a patient from hearing or understanding what you say. This frequently happens when words such as *cancer* or *heart surgery* frighten the patient so much that he fails to hear your message. When you see that a patient's frightened, don't go any further with your teaching. Wait until he starts asking questions—the signal that he's ready to hear more.

• ***Mistrust.*** A patient who shows signs of mistrust may be influenced by previous unpleasant experiences with hospitalization. He may also be mistrustful if he doesn't understand the roles of the many professionals involved in his care or if he receives conflicting infor-

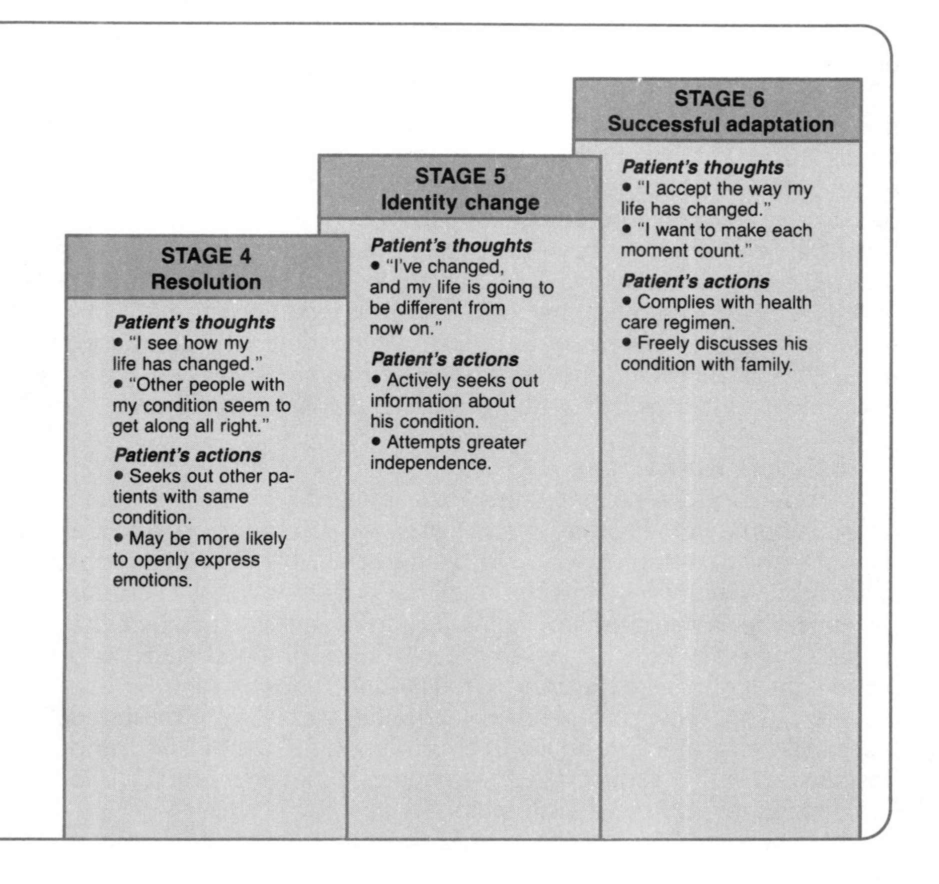

mation from them. For example, suppose you tell a patient during preoperative teaching that he'll be able to get up and walk the day after surgery, but his doctor tells him that he'll be allowed to get out of bed only to go to the bathroom. This discrepancy can be extremely upsetting for the patient. It can foster feelings of mistrust that may interfere with both your ability to teach and the patient's readiness to learn.

Stage of adaptation

A patient may go through various stages before successfully adapting to his illness, including disbelief, developing awareness, reorganization, resolution, and identity change. (See *Assessing Your Patient's Stage of Adaptation,* page 36.) Most patients don't progress in an orderly way from one stage to the next: a patient may skip one or two stages or regress to an earlier stage during a health crisis. During your assessment, be aware of the patient's stage of adaptation. This will help you understand his coping strategies, so you can avoid teaching him something he's not ready to learn. For example, suppose you're assessing a teen-aged patient whose neck was broken when he was thrown from a horse. The patient tells you what the doctor's said about his condition: he'll probably be permanently paralyzed from the neck down. But when you try to talk with him about rehabilitation, he responds by talking about going back to school and riding his horse again. This patient isn't ready to learn about rehabilitation; he hasn't accepted his condition.

A patient who denies his condition presents a paradoxical problem: you need to discuss the reality of his condition with him, but he isn't ready to acknowledge it. When a patient denies his condition, respect his response as a necessary coping mechanism. Then, gradually begin to talk with him about realistic plans for the future.

Emotional maturity

When you assess a patient's emotional maturity, try to determine his *developmental level* and his *self-esteem.* These factors affect a patient's ability to make decisions, take responsibility for their consequences, and manage his life—hallmarks of emotional maturity.

• ***Determine developmental level.*** Try to determine whether the patient has mastered the tasks of each developmental stage he's passed through. (See *Relating Growth and Development to Assessment Concerns,* pages 40-43.) Whether or not he's mastered these tasks can affect his ability to cope with the stress of illness and hospitalization. To reduce stress, a patient sometimes regresses to less difficult levels he's already passed.

Also recognize developmental tasks that are in a state of transition or stagnation. These tasks can affect a patient's readiness to learn by influencing his motivation to try out new behaviors. For instance, suppose your patient is a 15-year-old boy with insulin-dependent diabetes. Self-consciousness about his appearance and a desire to be "one of the gang"—typical adolescent concerns—may make it difficult for him to accept the change in body image his diabetes produces. Nevertheless, before your patient leaves the hospital, you'll need to teach him how to give himself insulin injections. But you know he may not be ready to learn the procedure because it sets him apart from his peers—one of the major fears of adolescence. Knowing your patient's developmental level helps you plan teaching strategies that compensate. For example, because adolescents develop their identity in relation to their peers and in opposition to their parents, this patient's readiness to learn self-injection techniques may improve if you conduct your teaching without his parents present.

• ***Assess self-esteem.*** A patient's self-esteem—his judgment of how he rates as a person—influences how he responds psychologically to illness. If a patient considers himself to be a good person, he can adapt to illness with an intact ego and will more likely be ready to learn. On the other hand, a patient who views himself as bad or worthless may feel overwhelmed by his illness and will less likely be ready to learn.

Past life experiences

As a person matures, he acquires certain skills and experiences that help prepare him for learning new tasks. A patient's experiences—not only with health care procedures but also with hobbies or work-related activities—can increase his readiness to learn by making learning more meaningful and familiar. For example, suppose you need to teach a patient how to apply adhesive paste around his ileostomy. If he's ever performed a task that required a similar skill—such as caulking a window—he'll be ready to learn this new task sooner than if he weren't familiar with the technique.

Patient and family goals

The goals of the patient and his family determine the patient's priorities for learning. Realistic goals can motivate a patient to learn, but "impossible dreams"—expectations beyond the patient's current capabilities—can discourage him in his efforts to learn.

• ***Recognize the patient's goals.*** The first step in recognizing the patient's learning goals is to discover what, if anything, he wants to know. Until the patient meets his goals, he'll be unable to meet the expectations of his family or the health care team. Similarly, a patient

RELATING GROWTH AND DEVELOPMENT TO ASSESSMENT CONCERNS

INFANT
Trust vs. mistrust

DEVELOPMENTAL TASKS
- Develops attachment to primary care giver
- Develops awareness of self as separate person
- Begins developing communication skills

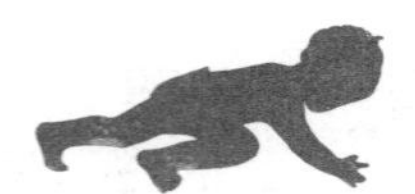

WHAT TO ASK
- Does the infant respond to the physical presence of his parents?
- How does he communicate his needs and feelings?

WHAT TO LOOK FOR
- Shows distress when family leaves
- Uses motor and verbal skills to communicate needs and feelings

TODDLER
Autonomy vs. shame and doubt

DEVELOPMENTAL TASKS
- Develops sense of autonomy
- Further develops sense of self
- Begins developing socialization skills

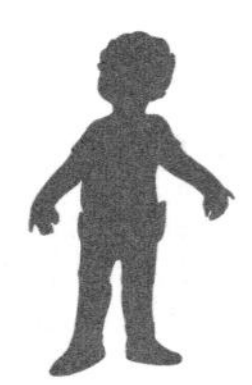

WHAT TO ASK
- Does the toddler prefer certain foods or activities?
- How does he acknowledge parental distress or approval?
- Does he play with other children or adults?

WHAT TO LOOK FOR
- Willing to follow whims
- Plays alongside others or interacts with them
- Approaches others with show-and-tell items

can't concentrate on learning if other goals are more important to him. Consider this example: a man in his early sixties undergoes a bowel resection for colon cancer, has complications, and faces prolonged hospitalization. His doctor encourages him to increase his activity to prevent further complications. His nurse wants him to take a more active role in learning, so he can become self-sufficient. His wife urges him to cooperate, so he can come home as soon as possible: she's worried about shouldering his responsibilities while he's hospitalized. But the patient's apathetic about learning self-care

PRESCHOOLER
Initiative vs. guilt

DEVELOPMENTAL TASKS
- Develops sense of purpose
- Masters self-care skills
- Develops sense of self, gender, identity, and family relationship

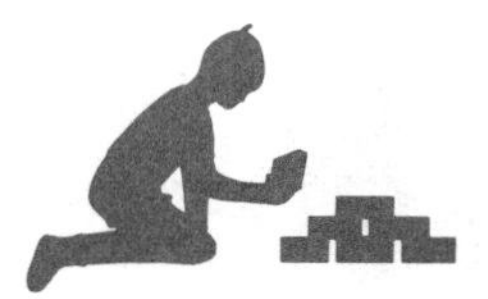

WHAT TO ASK
- Which self-care skills does the child perform at home?
- How does he keep busy at home?
- What's his reaction to schedules and routines?
- What would the child like to be when he grows up?
- What's his favorite activity?
- Can he state his name and identify family members?

WHAT TO LOOK FOR
- Occupies free time independently
- Participates in self-care activities
- Evaluates disapproval of others
- Initiates activities rather than just imitating others' actions

SCHOOL-AGE CHILD
Industry vs. inferiority

DEVELOPMENTAL TASKS
- Further develops sense of self through achievement
- Develops sense of right and wrong
- Shows more interaction with peers

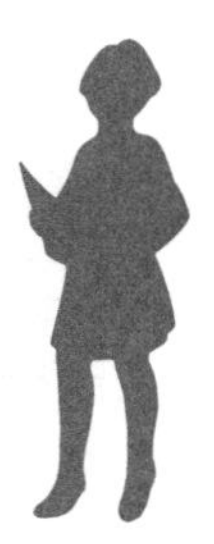

WHAT TO ASK
- What does the child do best?
- What's his favorite subject in school?
- Who's his best friend? What kinds of things do they do together?
- What would he do if he found a lost item in the playground?

WHAT TO LOOK FOR
- Talks about friends, family, and activities
- Interacts with others and initiates conversation
- Participates in self-care activities
- Attempts to improve his skills

(continued)

procedures. Why? There are several possible answers: first of all, he probably feels overwhelmed by the expectations of those involved in his care. Second, he may feel that he hasn't received enough information to make decisions about his future or to take positive action. And finally, he may be using all of his energy to meet his own immediate goal—survival.

When a patient feels overwhelmed by the goals others have set for him, he may react with frustration, anger, or even despair—barriers to effective learning. To help avoid this, you'll need to assess

RELATING GROWTH AND DEVELOPMENT TO ASSESSMENT CONCERNS *(continued)*

ADOLESCENT
Identity vs. role confusion

DEVELOPMENTAL TASKS
- Establishes self-identity
- Prepares for independent role in society
- Continues to develop relationships with peers of both sexes

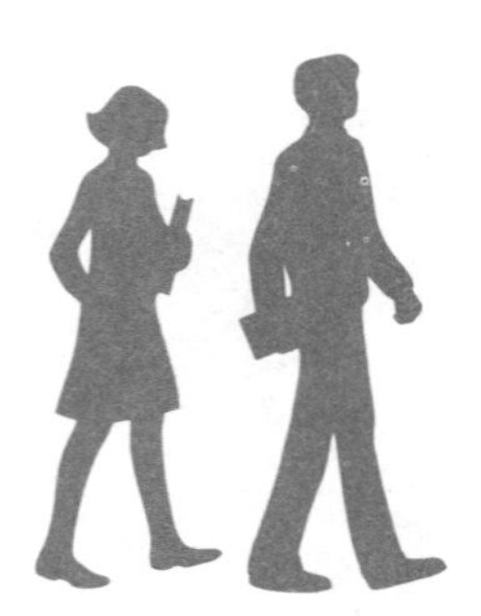

WHAT TO ASK
- Is he in school? Does he want to attend college or learn a trade?
- Who are his friends? Will they be visiting or calling while he's hospitalized?

WHAT TO LOOK FOR
- Expresses individuality through appearance or activities
- Interacts with significant peers and hospital staff
- Willing, if able, to continue school work

YOUNG ADULT
Intimacy vs. isolation

DEVELOPMENTAL TASKS
- Establishes independence from parental figures
- Initiates a permanent life-style
- Adjusts to companionship style
- Integrates values into career and socioeconomic constraints

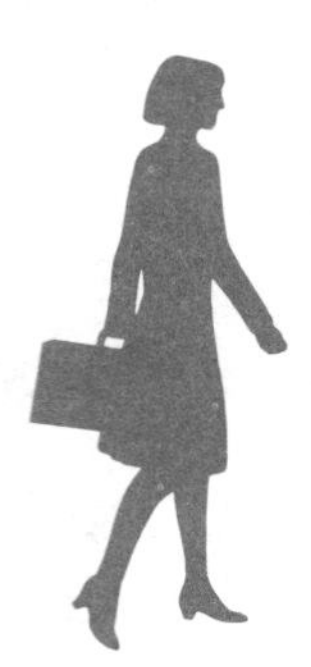

WHAT TO ASK
- Does he live at home with his parents? Or does he have his own family?
- Is he employed or in school?

WHAT TO LOOK FOR
- Forms role-appropriate relationships with staff and others
- Copes with hospital regulations
- Assists and directs care
- Forms intimate relationship with another person

his goals accurately and to share your information with his family and health care team. After you've determined what the patient's ready to learn, work with him, his family, and other members of the health care team to set realistic teaching goals.

• ***Recognize the family's goals.*** Does the patient's family have confidence in his ability to achieve his learning goals? Or do they believe he'll never be able to learn a particular skill or concept? Families often have expectations of what the hospitalized family member should accomplish. Are their goals realistic? If so, their

MIDDLE-AGED ADULT
Generativity vs. stagnation

DEVELOPMENTAL TASKS
- Establishes socioeconomic status
- Helps younger and older persons
- Finds satisfaction through his work, as a citizen and family member, or as a care provider

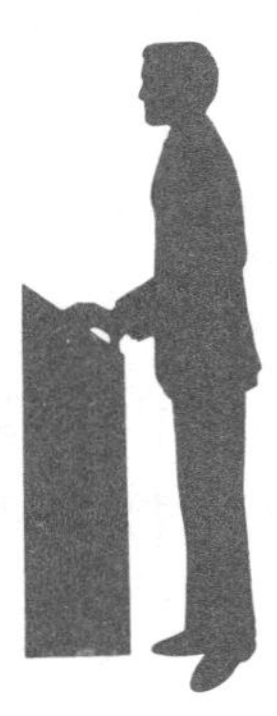

WHAT TO ASK
- What's the most satisfying thing in his life?
- Who are the important people in his life?
- Is he active in community affairs?

WHAT TO LOOK FOR
- Copes with hospital regulations
- Directs and participates in care

OLDER ADULT
Integrity vs. despair

DEVELOPMENTAL TASKS
- Forms mutually supportive relationships with grown children
- Adjusts to change in or loss of friends and relatives
- Prepares for retirement
- Uses leisure time in satisfying way
- Adapts to aging

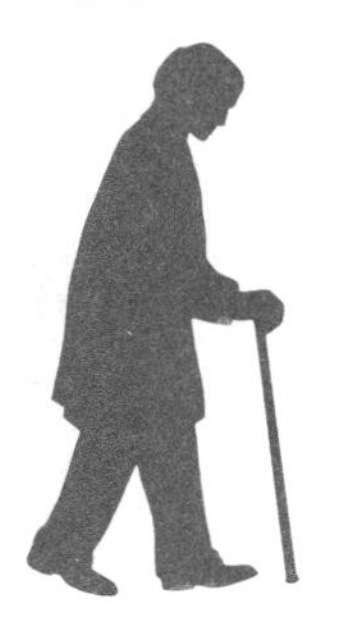

WHAT TO ASK
- Does he have any financial concerns?
- What are his retirement plans?
- What does he do in his leisure time?
- Does he have friends his own age?
- How does he feel about getting older?

WHAT TO LOOK FOR
- Shows concern for children and grandchildren
- Keeps current on world events
- Forms adult relationships with hospital staff
- Participates in care and decision making

support can increase the patient's readiness to learn. If not, their unrealistic expectations can make the patient feel uneasy or hesitant about learning.

The family's goals also reveal their willingness to take an active part in the learning process. Find out what they'd like to learn about the patient's illness. If the patient's family will be caring for him after he leaves the hospital, determine their goals for learning about home care procedures.

• ***Help the patient and his family set realistic goals.*** Many patients and families are unfamiliar or uncomfortable with goal setting. You can ease the process by asking them well-focused questions and by encouraging them to discuss their expectations with you as well as among themselves.

Encourage the patient and his family to develop goals geared toward the patient's true capabilities. For example, suppose your patient's had a cerebrovascular accident (CVA), with resulting right-sided hemiplegia. In this situation, a realistic goal might be to learn to walk with a cane. But, if your patient's had a total T6 spinal transection, such a goal would be impossible. Instead, a realistic long-term goal might be to learn how to function independently while using a wheelchair.

Working with both the patient and his family, write down their goals. Remember, each patient will achieve his goals at his own pace, so avoid setting an inflexible time limit for when he should learn a particular skill or concept. Otherwise, he may feel unnecessarily frustrated or depressed if he fails to meet the schedule. If possible, leave the list of goals with the patient and his family so they can review them, make changes, and set new priorities as the patient's condition changes.

Assessing willingness to learn

A patient becomes willing to learn when he recognizes a gap between what he knows and what he wants to know. Conversely, if a patient doesn't want to learn about and comply with a particular health care regimen, he won't—especially if it means giving up long-held habits without any evident reward. For example, an overweight diabetic patient who "feels fine" may be unwilling to learn and follow a modified diet to control his illness.

During your assessment, try to determine the patient's attitude about the subject you're planning to teach. Does he think this information is important for him to learn, or does he consider it a waste of time? Also consider the patient's health beliefs, sociocultural background, and religious beliefs—factors that can affect his willingness to learn by influencing his attitude toward health and illness.

Health beliefs

A patient's health beliefs determine his response to illness or the threat of illness. For example, a patient who says, "A yearly checkup is important to me," may believe his actions can help prevent certain health problems. His health beliefs tend to increase his willingness to learn. Another patient who says, "I'm afraid to see my doctor; he might find that something's wrong with me," may believe that his actions can have a negative effect by forcing him to confront a condition that frightens or confuses him.

By assessing your patient's health beliefs, you can determine how he makes health care decisions and predict his compliance with the treatment plan—essential information for planning an effective teaching strategy. (See *How Health Beliefs Affect Willingness to Learn.*) Generally, a patient's willingness to learn increases if he believes he's susceptible to a specific illness or that the illness would

HOW HEALTH BELIEFS AFFECT WILLINGNESS TO LEARN

Research shows that a patient learns better when he wants to learn. That's why it's important to assess your patient's health beliefs—they often reveal what he wants, or is willing, to learn. Knowing his health beliefs helps you predict his response to illness or the threat of illness, so you can tailor your teaching plan to meet his needs. In the chart below, an example illness—breast cancer—helps clarify how health beliefs affect a patient's willingness to learn.

PATIENT'S STATEMENT	PATIENT'S HEALTH BELIEF	NURSE'S ASSESSMENT
"I worry a lot about getting breast cancer. It runs in my family."	Believes in greater than average likelihood of getting breast cancer.	Patient's perceived *suscepti-bility* to breast cancer increases her willingness to learn about it.
"If I had breast cancer, my whole life would change."	Believes that breast cancer would affect all aspects of her life.	Patient's perception of the *seriousness* of breast cancer and its impact on her life increases her willingness to learn preventive measures and early treatments.
"Breast self-examinations can help me find lumps in my breasts."	Believes that breast self-examination is a helpful and important self-care procedure.	Patient's perception of the *benefit* of the procedure increases her willingness to learn and perform it.
"I don't have time to perform a breast self-examination each month."	Believes that performing breast self-examination would create burdensome life-style changes.	Patient's perception that the procedure would interfere with her routine indicates a *barrier* that may decrease her willingness to learn it.

have a serious effect on his life-style. In addition, if a patient believes his actions can prevent the illness or that taking action is less dangerous than incurring the illness, he'll be more willing to learn about and comply with the treatment plan.

- ***Assess locus of control.*** A patient's perception of his ability to bring about change—his *locus of control*—often determines his health beliefs. During your assessment, try to find out how the patient feels about his condition. Generally, a patient who believes he's in control of his illness is more willing to learn than a patient who feels powerless to alter it.
- ***Examine health practices.*** During your assessment, find out where the patient gets most of his health information and how he puts this information to use. A person's health practices often reflect his health beliefs. For example, a patient may include high-fiber foods in his diet if he believes this can help reduce the risk of colorectal cancer. Another patient may believe he can ward off arthritis by wearing a copper bracelet or drinking an herbal preparation.

Keep in mind that many people follow the advice of nonprofessionals—neighbors, relatives, friends—to treat illness. A patient who distrusts established medicine or uses folk remedies may be unwilling to learn about traditional treatments. To help this patient respond openly to your assessment questions, find out what nontraditional remedies he's been using. When you plan your teaching strategy, try to combine these nontraditional remedies with his prescribed regimen (provided, of course, that they don't interfere with legitimate medical and nursing care). For example, a patient could wear a copper bracelet while also taking prescribed medications.

Sociocultural background

From one generation to the next, families pass on specific values, beliefs, and customs that help determine how their members react to various circumstances. In many cultures, for example, women are more free to express their emotions than men. Ask your patient about his sociocultural background: where were his parents or ancestors born? How long has his family lived in this country? Does he speak a second language at home?

During your assessment, consider how the patient's sociocultural background has shaped his response to illness. For example, suppose your hypertensive patient is a 55-year-old American man whose parents immigrated to the United States from Ireland. In this patient's family, men are expected to present a strong, rugged image—a factor that may influence his willingness to learn the relaxation techniques his doctor prescribes.

When you assess a patient's sociocultural background, try to determine its impact on his current life-style. Does he still hold the values and customs of his ethnic group? If not, what changes has he made? Usually, the impact is less dramatic when several generations separate a patient from his family's country of origin.

• ***Avoid stereotyping.*** If you're familiar with accepted behavior within your patient's sociocultural group, you can assess his learning needs with greater insight. At the same time, however, you must remember that each patient is an individual, not a stereotype. Contrary to popular belief, for example, not all Italian-Americans are highly emotional, and not all Americans of Anglo-Saxon origin are stoic. Despite cultural influences, each patient is unique—and so is his response to learning.

Religious beliefs

A patient's religion can also affect his willingness to learn by influencing his attitudes toward illness and traditional medicine. For example, a patient who regards his CVA as a test of his faith or a divine punishment for wrongdoing may be unwilling to learn about rehabilitation techniques.

During your assessment, determine the nature and strength of your patient's religious beliefs. Does he have any religious beliefs about treating illness? Many Christian Scientists, for example, shun traditional medical treatment, believing that a person can cure illness by altering his thought processes. What role does religion play in the patient's daily routine? If his religion prohibits certain foods, for example, he may resist learning about dietary changes that conflict with his beliefs. By trying to accommodate the patient's religious beliefs and practices in your teaching plan, you can increase his willingness to learn and comply. (See *Reviewing Religious Beliefs and Practices,* pages 48 and 49.)

Assessing ability to learn

A patient's ability to learn depends on his current physical and mental status. Generally, a patient who is physically and mentally able to learn can master the skills and understanding necessary to manage his health problems. On the other hand, a patient who has a physical or mental deficit—such as a disabling illness or severe stress—may be temporarily or permanently unable to do so.

REVIEWING RELIGIOUS BELIEFS AND PRACTICES

RELIGION	BIRTH AND DEATH RITUALS	DIETARY RESTRICTIONS	PRACTICES IN HEALTH CRISIS
Adventist (Advent Christian Church, Seventh-Day Adventist, Church of God)	None (baptism of adults only)	Alcohol, coffee, tea, narcotics, and stimulants prohibited; in many groups, meat prohibited also	Communion and baptism performed. Some members believe in divine healing, anointing with oil, and prayer. Some regard Saturday as Sabbath.
Baptist (27 different groups)	At birth, none (baptism of believers only); before death, counseling by clergy and prayer	Alcohol prohibited; in some groups, coffee and tea prohibited also	Some believe in healing by laying on of hands. Resistance to medical therapy occasionally approved.
Church of Christ	None (baptism at age 8 or older)	Alcohol discouraged	Communion, anointing with oil, laying on of hands, and counseling by minister.
Church of Christ, Scientist (Christian Scientist)	At birth, none; before death, counseling by Christian Science practitioner	Alcohol, coffee, and tobacco prohibited	Many members refuse all treatment, including drugs, biopsies, physical examination, and transfusions. Vaccination only when required by law. Alteration of thoughts believed to cure illness. Hypnotism and psychotherapy prohibited. (Christian Science nursing homes honor these beliefs.)
Church of Jesus Christ of Latter-day Saints (Mormon)	At birth, none (baptism at age 8 or older); before death, baptism and gospel preaching	Alcohol, tobacco, tea, and coffee prohibited; meat intake limited	Divine healing through the laying on of hands; communion on Sunday; some members may refuse treatment. Many wear special undergarment.
Eastern Orthodox Churches (Albanian, Bulgarian, Cypriot, Czechoslovakian, Egyptian, Greek, Polish, Romanian, Russian, Syrian, Turkish)	At birth, baptism and confirmation; before death, last rites. For members of the Russian Orthodox Church, arms are crossed after death, fingers set in cross, and unembalmed body clothed in natural fiber.	For members of the Russian Orthodox Church and usually the Greek Orthodox Church, no meat or dairy products on Wednesday, Friday, and during Lent.	Anointing of the sick. For members of the Russian Orthodox Church, cross necklace replaced immediately after surgery and no shaving of male patients except in preparation for surgery. For members of the Greek Orthodox Church, communion and Sacrament of Holy Unction.
Episcopalian	At birth, baptism; before death, occasional last rites	For some members, abstention from meat on Friday, fasting before communion (which may be received daily)	Communion, prayer, and counseling by minister.

Note: Because religious beliefs may vary within particular sects, individual practices may differ from those described here.

RELIGION	BIRTH AND DEATH RITUALS	DIETARY RESTRICTIONS	PRACTICES IN HEALTH CRISIS
Islam (Muslim)	If abortion occurs before 130 days, fetus treated as discarded tissue; after 130 days, as a human being. Before death, confession of sins with family present; after death, only relatives or friends may touch the body.	Pork prohibited; daylight fasting during ninth month of Islamic calendar	Faith healing for the patient's morale only; conservative members reject medical therapy.
Jehovah's Witnesses	None	Abstention from foods to which blood has been added	Generally, no blood transfusion; may require court order for emergency transfusion.
Judaism	Ritual circumcision after birth; burial of dead fetus; ritual washing of dead; burial (including organs and other body tissues) occurs as soon as possible; no autopsy	For Orthodox and Conservative Jews, kosher dietary laws (for example, pork and shellfish prohibited); for Reform Jews, usually no restrictions	Donation or transplantation of organs requires rabbinical consultation. For Orthodox and Conservative Jews, medical procedures may be prohibited on Sabbath—from sundown Friday to sundown Saturday—and on special holidays.
Lutheran	Baptism usually performed 6 to 8 weeks after birth	None	Communion, prayer, and counseling by minister.
Orthodox Presbyterian	Infant baptism; scripture reading and prayer before death	None	Communion, prayer, and counseling by minister.
Pentecostal (Assembly of God, Foursquare Church)	None (baptism only after age of accountability)	Abstention from alcohol, tobacco, meat slaughtered by strangling, any food to which blood has been added, and sometimes pork	Divine healing through prayer, anointing with oil, and laying on of hands.
Roman Catholic	Infant baptism, including baptism of aborted fetus without sign of clinical death (tissue necrosis); before death, anointing of the sick	Fasting or abstention from meat on Ash Wednesday and on Fridays during Lent; this practice usually waived for the hospitalized	Burial of major amputated limb (sometimes) in consecrated ground; donation or transplantation of organs allowed if benefit to recipient is proportional to the donor's potential harm.
United Methodist	None (baptism of children and adults only)	None	Communion before surgery or similar crisis; donation of body parts encouraged.

During your assessment, focus on examining the patient's current status. Does he have any problems that could interfere with his ability to learn? Assess his physical condition, intellectual level, and preferred learning style. Also consider his support system and socioeconomic status—factors that could affect his ability to learn by causing or reducing stress.

Physical condition

Examine the patient for any physiologic barriers to learning. For example, a patient's likely to be unresponsive to your teaching if

THE HOME ENVIRONMENT: KEY TO COMPLIANCE

One of the biggest frustrations of patient teaching occurs when a patient learns a self-care procedure in the hospital but doesn't comply with it at home. How can you help prevent this? By considering your patient's home environment when you assess his learning needs. This illustration shows some common examples of factors that may influence compliance.

Do friends, neighbors, or community organizations provide adequate support?
Is his home environment safe? For example, does he have a smoke alarm and a fire extinguisher?
Does the patient have a good support system at home? For example, do family members meet his physical needs?
Does his home have modern plumbing and electricity?

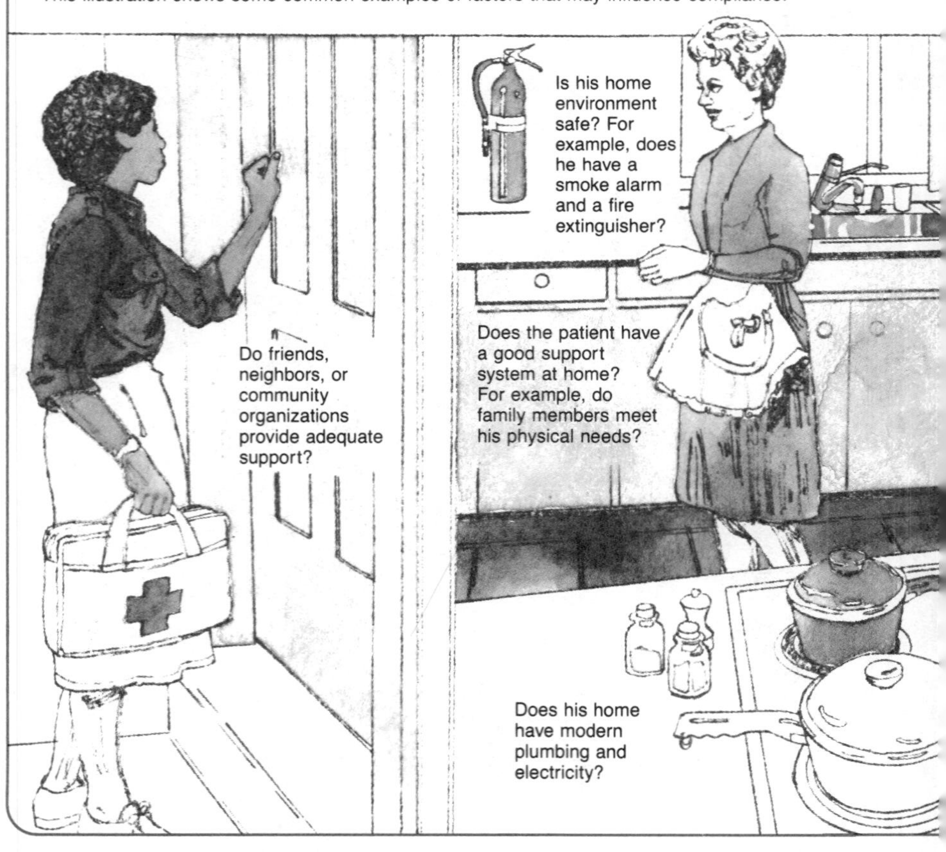

he's in pain. A patient who's fatigued or weak may find it difficult or impossible to respond fully to your teaching. Similarly, fever, nausea, or vomiting can make a patient temporarily unable to learn.

A *sensory-impaired* patient will probably need teaching sessions aimed at his unimpaired senses. During your assessment, explore the extent of his deficit and his method of compensating for it. If the patient has a hearing loss, for example, find out whether he uses a hearing aid, whether his deafness is unilateral or bilateral, whether he can lip-read, and whether he can speak. This information not only allows you to plan an effective teaching strategy but also

If you can identify barriers to compliance before you teach, you can modify your teaching plan to overcome them. The result? Not only will your patient be more likely to comply but your teaching will be easier.

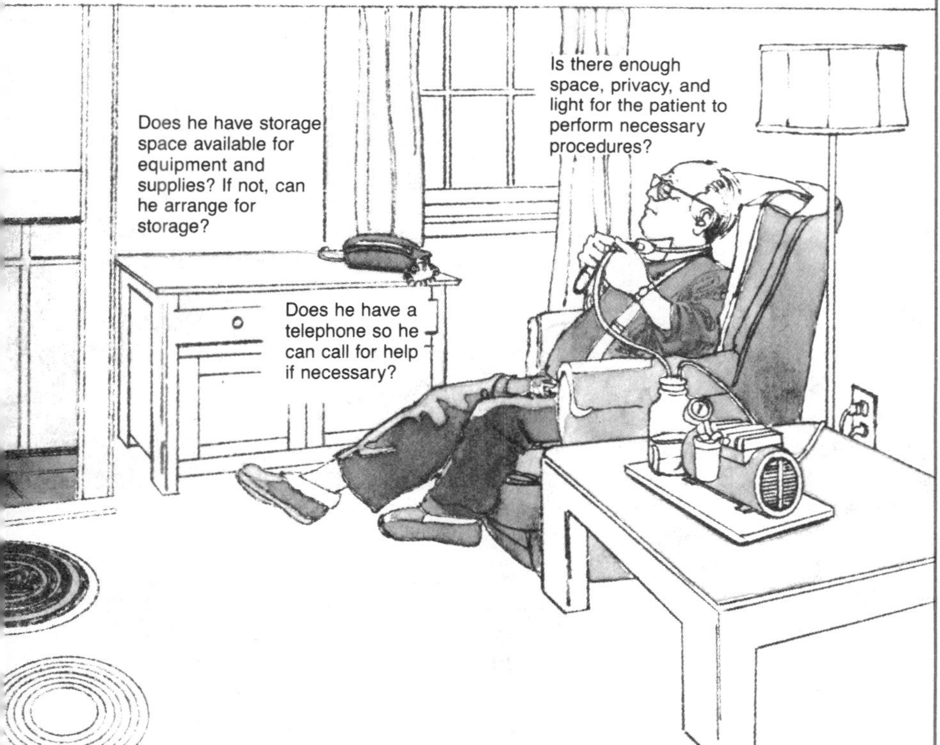

helps you to complete your assessment.

A *physically handicapped* patient may be unable to learn certain skills. If your patient has rheumatoid arthritis, for example, he may be unable to perform self-care procedures that require precise hand movements. However, he may still overcome his disability if he's strongly motivated.

A patient's reaction to the *stress of hospitalization* can create or heighten barriers to learning. When you assess your patient's physical condition, consider the following barriers:

• ***Sensory underload and overload.*** Some patients experience an overall lack of stimulation—*sensory underload*—while in the hospital. For example, a patient who's on bed rest won't receive the variety of stimulation available to an ambulatory patient. Other patients experience a heightened state of sensory awareness—a condition called *sensory overload.* This results when a patient perceives sensations more intensely than normal or when he receives sensory input simultaneously from a variety of sources.

Sensory underload and overload produce similar effects—among the most common are anxiety, restlessness, decreased attention span, and somnolence. Both can interfere with the patient's ability to learn by causing confusion and affecting his receptivity to teaching.

• ***Disorientation.*** Remember to evaluate your patient's orientation to time, person, and place—even if his condition doesn't normally warrant such an assessment. A hospitalized patient often experiences some disorientation—possibly resulting from the unfamiliar surroundings. This blocks learning because a disoriented patient can't think quickly or coherently. So remain alert for signs of disorientation while you're assessing or teaching the patient. The clue may be a vague expression or a look of fear. In a few patients, signs include anger and refusal to cooperate.

• ***Sleep deprivation.*** A common effect of hospitalization, sleep deprivation saps a patient's ability to learn. Assess your patient for fatigue, muscle weakness, malaise, or apathy—possible indications of sleep deprivation. A patient who also seems irritable, suspicious, or confused may be deprived of rapid eye movement sleep—the type needed for mental well-being.

• ***Pain.*** The anxiety of hospitalization often heightens a patient's response to pain, which can hinder his ability to learn by disrupting his concentration and causing fatigue. Be sure to assess your patient for pain before you attempt to teach him. Also check for nonverbal expressions of pain, such as grimacing, unusual posture or body position, or nervousness. Remember that some patients respond to pain with increased activity.

IS YOUR PATIENT'S FAMILY INTERFERING?

Your patient's relationship with his family can make learning easier—or more difficult. Properly directed, family members can greatly improve a patient's willingness and ability to learn. But when family members upset your patient, create stress, or undermine your teaching efforts, learning suffers. How can you tell if your patient's family is interfering? These behaviors may be telltale signs.

HOW YOUR PATIENT ACTS

- Refuses to see his family or asks that no one be allowed to visit
- Argues with his family or shows anger toward them
- Experiences signs of stress, such as tachycardia, agitation, perspiration, or flushed skin, when his family visits
- Becomes depressed, uncooperative, or aggressive.

HOW HIS FAMILY ACTS

- Doesn't visit the patient or doesn't interact with him during visits
- Argues with the patient or shows anger toward him
- Avoids physical contact with the patient
- Contradicts your teaching or encourages the patient not to cooperate.

If your patient suffers from chronic pain, assess his ability to cope. Over time, a patient with chronic pain may develop coping mechanisms that permit him to continue functioning but that also interfere with learning. For example, a patient who can't control his pain may compensate by attempting to control his environment and could become manipulative or uncooperative.

Intellectual status

A patient must have adequate intelligence to learn. Of course, your assessment of his intellectual status won't be definitive, but it should determine his basic abilities and identify potential barriers to learning.

• ***Estimate intelligence.*** You can estimate a patient's intelligence by the vocabulary and language skills he uses, the amount of detail with which he describes his illness, and the extent to which he recalls past events. In addition, you can estimate his intelligence by assessing his understanding and compliance with past medical instructions. Note the extent of his schooling, such as the highest grade completed and courses of study taken. Also note what type of job the patient has.

Conversations with the patient may also reveal his ability to understand abstract or concrete ideas and to solve problems. To determine if the patient understands what you're saying, ask him to repeat—in his own words—what you've said. The patient's responses to questions involving general knowledge may provide additional insight.

Keep in mind that a patient's apparently limited intellectual functioning may be caused by disorientation. Of course, a patient who is critically ill or has a language barrier may also be unable to participate actively in learning.

• ***Consider learning barriers.*** Check the patient's chart for information about any learning disabilities, such as dyslexia, or language disorders, such as aphasia. If you plan to use written instructions to teach the patient, be sure to assess his literacy. Also check for such conditions as mental retardation or senility, which will directly affect ability to learn. If your patient's mentally retarded, he may be able to learn skills but probably won't be able to understand concepts or become proficient in decision making. A senile patient usually isn't receptive to teaching and learns poorly, if at all. When assessing a patient with either of these barriers, be sure to explore your own feelings; don't let them affect your impression of the patient's learning abilities.

Learning style

A patient's ability to learn increases when teaching incorporates his preferred learning style. During your assessment, try to determine if your patient's primarily a visual learner, a tactile learner, or an auditory learner. (See Chapter 1 for more information on learning styles.)

The support system

A patient can receive emotional support from a variety of sources—including family, friends, the community, and church or religious groups. Together, these sources comprise a patient's *support system*—the group he turns to for comfort, aid, and information to help him cope with life. Having a strong support system reduces stress and may raise a patient's self-confidence and self-esteem, allowing him to concentrate on learning.

During your assessment, explore the nature and adequacy of the patient's support system. Observe how *family* members talk with the patient and with each other, and note who they turn to, among themselves, for guidance and emotional support. Do they seem to communicate openly and to respect each other's feelings and opinions? Observing the interaction between the patient and his family may give you clues to his role and responsibilities in the family and

CHECKLIST

WHAT TO ASSESS

- ☐ The patient's current emotional state
- ☐ His stage of adaptation to illness
- ☐ His emotional maturity
- ☐ His developmental stage
- ☐ His self-image
- ☐ His past life experiences
- ☐ His learning goals—and his family's
- ☐ The patient's health beliefs
- ☐ His sociocultural background
- ☐ His religious beliefs
- ☐ His physical condition
- ☐ His intellectual status
- ☐ His learning style
- ☐ His socioeconomic status
- ☐ Family support system and availability of support groups

to the strength and character of his relationships with family members.

Ask the patient about his *friendships,* and note which of his friends visit him during his hospitalization. Does he seem to get along better or talk more freely with his friends than with certain family members?

Also assess the patient's reliance on *community services,* such as independent health care providers, community agencies, and self-help groups. Has the patient rejected any resources that are available to him? If so, why?

Finally, assess the patient's reliance on *church or religious groups.* Such groups may provide the patient with much-needed comfort and support after he leaves the hospital.

Socioeconomic status

During your assessment, be sure to consider your patient's socioeconomic status. After all, research shows that patients with higher incomes suffer less anxiety about hospitalization, and so are better able to learn, than those with lower incomes. A patient who's financially secure tends to view illness more as a minor inconvenience than as a major disruption of his life and livelihood. This patient often has job security, good health insurance coverage, and easy access to appropriate health care. For all of these reasons, he's less threatened by pain and illness than is a patient with a lower income. This increases his sense of control over his condition and, as a result, improves his ability to learn.

THE OUTCOME

By assessing your patient before you begin teaching, you can identify a wide range of factors that enhance or impede learning. Because assessment is characteristically an ongoing process, you'll be able to recognize how these factors change as your patient's condition changes.

After you've gathered your assessment data, you're then ready to formulate a "teaching diagnosis"—in effect, your evaluation of the patient's readiness, willingness, and ability to learn. Your teaching diagnosis, in turn, serves as the springboard for planning and implementing truly effective patient teaching.

3

Planning and teaching

Introduction

Having completed your assessment and identified your patient's learning needs, you're probably eager to get on with your teaching. Or perhaps you're a little nervous, wondering where you should begin. Whether you're eager or nervous, taking the time now to develop a well-thought-out teaching plan can facilitate your teaching and improve your skills.

Certainly no one has to convince you of the overwhelming importance of patient teaching. Most likely, you've been doing your share of teaching since your first day on nursing duty and have naturally become better and better at it. You may nevertheless tend to dismiss a teaching plan as an extra for which you have neither the time nor the need. This, however, would be a serious mistake.

Why develop a teaching plan?

As any good teacher will certainly tell you, planning lies at the root of effective teaching. Even though your planning probably won't be evident to your patient, it will make you seem organized, competent, and confident to him. That's important because a patient's impression of you as a teacher can greatly influence his willingness to learn and, thus, your teaching effectiveness.

Your attention to planning now, before you start to teach, may also result in one of those *spontaneous* interchanges between pupil and teacher that rests at the heart of the best teaching. What's more, a teaching plan has other proven advantages for you. For example, a teaching plan will simplify your actual teaching by providing a model you can follow so you don't constantly have to redirect your efforts. It will provide you with an objective basis for evaluating the patient's learning and allow you to get better results. A teaching plan will also save time for you and your colleagues.

When you veer from your teaching plan

Naturally, no matter how painstakingly you put together any teaching plan, you still may have to abbreviate and modify it when other demands impinge on your time. And sometimes, changes in the patient's condition or some other unforeseen circumstances may diminish the importance of following the plan. There will be times, also, when your plan is more honored in the breach.

Don't let the inevitability of veering from your teaching plan dissuade you from preparing one. Always keep in mind that the act of thinking through a formal, *ideal* plan is likely to enhance even the most impromptu bedside teaching session.

LEARNING ABOUT PLANNING

What's in a teaching plan?

Simply stated, a *teaching plan* is a carefully organized, written presentation of what the patient must learn and how you'll provide the instruction. It establishes the standards for later evaluating the results of your teaching. Broadly, it should be based on the patient's learning needs, as he's identified them and as you and other members of the health care team have pinpointed them. It should be undertaken in close collaboration with the patient, and it should be realistic enough for you to carry out during a short hospital stay. (Or it must include appropriate provisions for follow-up home teaching.) It should also allow you to be flexible in your teaching and to accommodate the demands of hospital life, such as a patient's sleepless night (which characteristically will make him unreceptive to your teaching the next day) or your limited time for teaching.

POLISHING YOUR TEACHING SKILLS

Your teaching skills, like any other skills you've acquired in nursing, can be refined with practice and direction. And that's especially important today with the growing emphasis on shorter hospital stays and cost containment. After all, effective and timely teaching can improve a patient's understanding of his condition and the prospects for his compliance with treatment. To improve your teaching skills, use these tips:

- Expand your knowledge base by reading professional publications, attending inservice and continuing-education programs, and maintaining a broad range of professional contacts.
- Ask your institution's staff development department to schedule inservice classes that can benefit your entire unit. Then follow up with conferences on your unit for more detailed discussion about what you learned.
- If you're not up to date on a subject you must teach, ask the staff development department to supply the names of specialists in that subject. Then call one for an appointment.
- Observe more experienced nurses while they're teaching patients. What makes their teaching effective? What kind of rapport do they have with their patients? How do they reach difficult-to-teach patients? Which of their methods could you use effectively?
- If you have a patient who's unusually difficult to teach, ask a colleague or a nursing consultant to do the teaching while you observe.
- Ask a colleague whom you consider an especially good teacher to sit in while you teach. Ask her to review your teaching tools and techniques and offer pointers for your next teaching session. If you're uncomfortable having a third person present while you teach, try role-playing the session beforehand; this can smooth any rough edges in your presentation and help put you at ease for the actual session.

Of the many types of teaching plans you'll come across, you'll probably have the most experience with these three: the standard teaching plan, developed by an institution or a commercial company for use with patients having similar learning needs; the individual teaching plan you yourself devise for a patient; and the cardex, which becomes a shorthand version of the plan's intent and content. The ready-made cardex and standard plans can be handy, time-saving resources, but they must always be adapted to your patient's specific needs.

While the scope of these plans differs, each should contain the same elements: a statement of the patient's learning goals, an outline of the content to be taught, a selection of teaching tools and methods, and some provision for evaluating the results.

Learning goals

When stating the patient's learning goals, make them specific enough so that other members of the health care team will readily understand what is to be taught, why it should be taught, and how it's to be evaluated. (See *Writing Learning Goals Clearly.*) State these goals in terms of patient behaviors that can be observed and can therefore indicate whether learning has taken place.

Be sure to consider the domains of learning when setting goals. Approached from this viewpoint, learning falls into three domains: the *cognitive,* dealing with tasks that primarily reflect thought processes; the *psychomotor,* dealing with learning in the physical and motor areas; and the *affective,* dealing with attitudes, expressions of feelings, and an individual's value system.

In much of what a patient learns, all three domains can be involved—although not equally. Let's say you're teaching a patient about subcutaneous injection sites. The cognitive task of identifying the site correctly will be primary. Also important will be the patient's use of the needle at the site, which is a psychomotor task. Lastly, his reaction to using the needle, which could be one of anxiety or lack of confidence, falls into the affective domain.

In the course of clarifying the patient's learning goals, take a moment to think about how you'll evaluate whether and what the patient has learned. Deciding at the outset what evaluation techniques, such as question-and-answer or return demonstration, will best reveal the patient's progress can help you find the precise words to phrase his learning goals. This is particularly true when you're establishing learning goals in the affective domain, because attitudes are difficult to measure behaviorally and learning in this domain generally takes place slowly over time. How, for example, can you be sure your patient has overcome his anxiety about subcutaneous

WRITING LEARNING GOALS CLEARLY

To clearly express your patient's learning goals, you'll need to focus on what aspects of his behavior you're aiming to change. His learning behaviors, and your goals for him, fall into the three learning domains: cognitive, psychomotor, and affective.

Your patient may have learning goals in all three domains. For example, understanding his dietary changes would fall into the cognitive domain, while complying with these changes would fall into the affective domain. Taking his blood pressure would fall into the psychomotor domain.

With these domains in mind, you can write clear and concise learning goals for your patient. These goals should clarify what you're going to teach, indicate the behavior you expect to see, and clearly set criteria for later evaluating how successfully the patient has learned.

Review the two sets of sample learning goals below for a patient with chronic renal failure. Notice that the goals in the well-phrased set start with a precise action verb, confine themselves to one task, and describe learning that is measurable and observable. In contrast, the poorly phrased goals may encompass many tasks. They also describe learning that is difficult or even impossible to measure.

WELL-PHRASED LEARNING GOALS	POORLY PHRASED LEARNING GOALS
Cognitive domain	
The patient with chronic renal failure will be able to:	
• state when to administer each drug. • describe symptoms of elevated blood pressure. • list allowed and prohibited foods on his diet.	• know his medication schedule. • know when his blood pressure is elevated. • realize his dietary restrictions.
Psychomotor domain	
The patient with chronic renal failure will be able to:	
• take his blood pressure accurately, using a stethoscope and a sphygmomanometer. • read a thermometer correctly. • collect a urine sample, using sterile technique.	• take his blood pressure. • use a thermometer. • bring in a urine sample for laboratory studies.
Affective domain	
The patient with chronic renal failure will be able to:	
• comply with dietary restrictions to maintain normal electrolyte values. • verbalize adjustments to be made in the home environment. • keep scheduled doctor appointments.	• appreciate the relationship of diet to renal failure. • adjust successfully to limitations imposed by chronic renal failure. • realize the importance of seeing his doctor regularly.

injections? Certainly, you could ask him if he still feels anxious. You could also assess his willingness to perform the procedure. Or you could observe for hesitation or signs of stress as he's doing it. By selecting evaluation techniques like these during your planning, you can formulate precise, measurable learning goals.

• ***Involve the patient in setting goals.*** Your teaching and the patient's learning are so intricately involved that sharing responsibility with him is essential if your teaching is to be effective. This mutuality begins with step one in your teaching plan—setting learning goals—and comes into play at each succeeding step. It might seem quicker and easier just to set down what you expect or wish your patient to achieve. But when you work closely with the patient to establish learning goals, you give him a chance to add his concerns and expectations to your professional expertise. This will promote co-operation and compliance with treatment.

You may need some practice at first in eliciting the patient's contributions. One technique you might find useful is the reflective method. For example, you might say to your patient with emphysema, "You seem concerned about your activity level and returning to work. How much energy does your job require?" Or, "As I see it, you want to know how to recognize when you're overextending yourself and what to do to recover. What signs have you noticed and what have you tried before?"

Content

The content of your teaching plan represents what you, the doctor, and the other members of the health care team determine the patient *needs* to know, blended with what the patient *wants* to know. Whether you're working with a ready-made or an individualized plan, you'll need to organize its content.

Start by recording your main points and then supply the detailed, supporting information for each point. Be sure to begin with simple concepts and work toward more complex ones. These cardinal principles of organization will prove especially helpful when you're teaching a patient with little education or one who doesn't learn well through listening.

Teaching methods

Most of your teaching will probably be done on a one-on-one basis, giving you an opportunity to learn about your patient, to build a relationship with him, and to tailor your teaching to his particular needs. But sometimes you'll need to teach a group of patients. First, a word about these situations. Group teaching works well when the patients have experienced, or are about to experience, a common medical situation. They may be facing the prospect of a mastectomy or recovering from a myocardial infarction.

Whatever the group's common experience, it usually results in some valuable pluses. Patients who share a condition tend to support and motivate one another. At times, they learn as much from each other as they do from you. From your point of view, teaching a group of patients obviously saves time for the nurses on your unit.

When you have the responsibility for helping a group develop a sense of identity and cohesiveness, take advantage of certain proven ways to make the group session more successful. (See *Setting the Stage for Successful Group Teaching,* page 64.)

Besides group teaching, other methods and tips for successful, efficient teaching are legion. But you may benefit from reviewing some of the more fundamental methods of teaching.

• ***Discussion.*** Whether used in individual or group teaching, discussion allows for the open exchange of ideas and information between you and your patient—rather than assuming that you have all the answers. As the discussion moves back and forth between you and the patient, the very act of asking questions or making comments involves the patient more actively in the problem-solving process: he begins, in a small, informal way, to take some responsibility for his own learning.

In addition, discussion can be a valuable follow-up to a lecture, a group-teaching session, or an audiovisual presentation.

• ***Demonstration, practice, and return demonstration.*** This technique, related to the show-and-tell in a child's classroom, is especially useful after a one-on-one discussion with your patient. There, you've set the stage for demonstrating a treatment or the use of equipment unfamiliar to the patient. Here, you demonstrate step-by-step, so your patient can imitate what you do. The demonstration can be impromptu, at the patient's bedside, or can be given during a scheduled teaching session. One isn't necessarily superior to the other. Your choice depends on the circumstances.

For instance, an impromptu demonstration is in order if an ostomy patient asks you to show him how to apply his pouch. He wants to know *now*—not later at the formal teaching demonstration you were planning. By taking time now to show him the correct procedure, you're also offering him support in a tense new situation.

A scheduled demonstration usually takes advance planning, since you'll want to be both knowledgeable and confident as you teach the patient. So assemble your materials in advance, and rehearse your presentation until you can convey an air of quiet authority to your patient.

After the demonstration, you'll want to give the patient time to practice, to "do it himself" in private—especially if the need for the procedure results from some major change in body maintenance or image, such as a colostomy.

If it seems advisable, provide the patient with a sheet of written guidelines to the steps he's learning. After allowing time for practice, reinforce your original demonstration with a review that gives the patient ample opportunity for active participation.

SETTING THE STAGE FOR SUCCESSFUL GROUP TEACHING

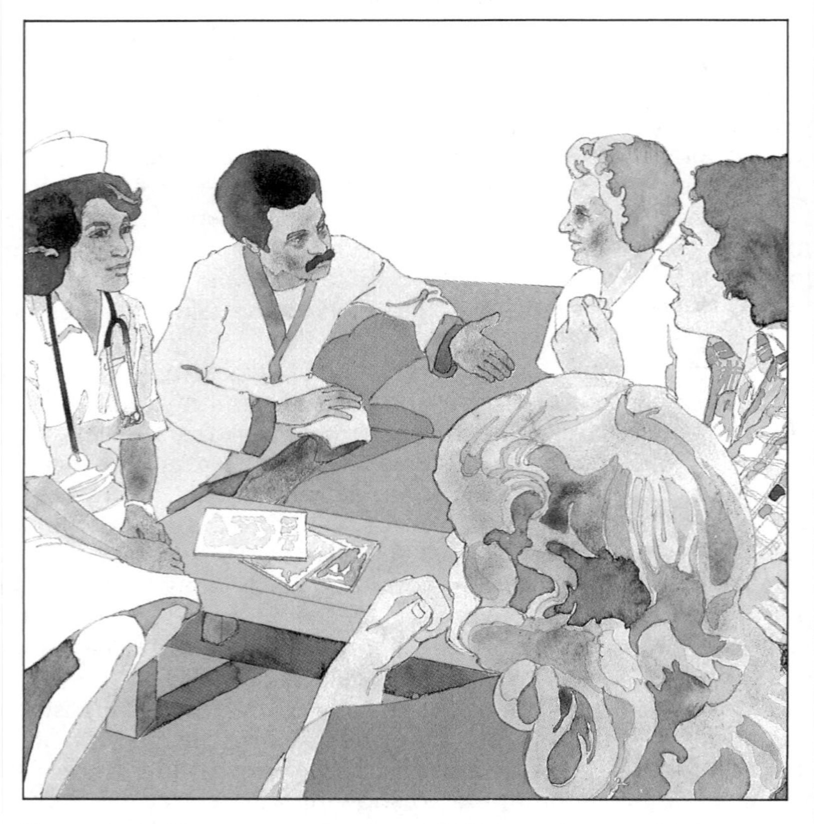

When you're teaching a group, you'll want to enhance the learning process by helping the patients develop a group identity and cohesiveness. Here are some useful techniques:

Shape the environment
- Hold the meeting at a round table, or arrange chairs in a circle. This increases interaction by making participants feel equal to each other and to the teacher.
- Limit the group to 5 to 7 patients to allow for maximum personal exchange and discussion.
- Check the temperature and lighting of the meeting room to be certain that neither is uncomfortable or distracting.
- Serve coffee, tea, or cold drinks to keep the atmosphere informal and relaxed.

Initiate discussion and maintain an overview
- Introduce yourself.
- Ask patients to introduce themselves and to share a bit of personal information.
- Explain the meeting's purpose.
- Invite the group to identify the meeting's goals and ground rules.
- Encourage everyone's participation and be gracious about allowing anyone to leave who isn't comfortable or doesn't wish to participate.
- Use a light rein, yet keep the group close to the agreed-upon areas for discussion.
- Act as a resource, providing information and clarification when necessary.
- Summarize at the end of the discussion, and lead the group to agree on what has been learned.

Occasionally, you'll encounter a patient who's resistant to, or uncomfortable with, such direct teaching methods. In that case, you'll have to work an abbreviated demonstration into your bedside care. This seemingly casual presentation can be drawn directly from your planned, full-scale demonstration; hence the need for careful planning in your teaching.

• ***Role playing.*** This teaching technique, which seems simple and spontaneous, becomes a powerful tool for learning. In role playing, your patient acts out an assigned but unrehearsed role in a hypothetical situation. In this way, he can prepare himself for a similar but real situation.

Role playing provides a safe environment in which to try out new behaviors or explore alternatives. The patient can take the opportunity to project himself into a situation that's likely to happen—and to plan ahead. If you have an adolescent patient who has just learned he has cancer, role playing can help him "practice" how to tell his friends and teachers about his illness and how to deal with their reactions. Role playing typically works best when a patient really puts himself into the part. He's then better able to transfer what he's learned from the imagined situation to the reality of his everyday life.

A follow-up discussion can enhance the benefits of the role-playing session if you guide the patient to examine his responses with such questions as "What was right about what you did?" "What was wrong?" "How did it feel?" "What would you do differently the next time?"

• ***Case study.*** A case study is a simulated situation, either written or spoken, very much like one the patient is currently facing. Using this approach, like using role playing, involves the patient in sample problem solving. However, the focus of the problem solving differs. Role playing casts the patient into a situation and emphasizes how he feels and responds in it. In a case study, the patient deals with the sample problem more objectively, as an observer and evaluator of someone else's behavior.

Your responsibility also varies slightly. In role playing, once you've established a situation, the patient more or less takes over, and the outcome is unpredictable. In a case study, you provide direct guidance through your questions and assistance. You might, for example, present your hypertensive patient with the case of a person with the same condition who's experiencing headaches and lack of energy. You'd ask your patient, "What could be causing his headaches?" "What can he do to alleviate them?" "At what point should he call his doctor?" Then you'd have him come up with possible courses of action for the case patient and weigh the pros and cons of each.

• ***Self-monitoring.*** In this teaching technique, the patient or his family—rather than you, as his nurse—becomes responsible for collecting the relevant data.

The patient who monitors himself ideally gains a heightened awareness of the aspects of his behavior or environment that call for correction. Let's say you have a patient with vascular headaches who begins to chart their occurrence and characterize the setting and emotional climate in which they occur. The patient might record that a headache began after eating a meal or drinking several glasses of wine, while in a stressful situation at home, or while in a smoke-filled conference room at work. His aim, of course, is to discover the factors that trigger his headaches so he can take corrective action.

The format for self-monitoring should encourage the patient to chart random factors that could prove significant, as well as the more accepted and acknowledged causative factors. Together, you and the patient decide the duration of self-monitoring. Once the patient has collected information for the agreed-upon period, you and he can then sift through what seem to be related or suspicious factors.

• ***Lecture.*** This traditional form of teaching is usually geared to larger groups of patients. A somewhat formal approach to teaching, a lecture is usually given in a classroom or conference room at a scheduled time. While lecturing seems like a logical means for conveying a large body of information to a group with similar concerns, it has serious drawbacks for patient teaching.

For the patient, the lecture is a passive form of learning. And since it depends almost solely upon language, it can shortchange patients with limited vocabulary or verbal skills or impaired hearing. Lecturing to patients for whom English is a second language is not usually a good teaching bet. And it has yet another drawback. As a one-way process for delivering information, lecturing can lead to misunderstanding and misinterpretation. And you may not discover the problem until it surfaces later in some medical complication.

If you do find yourself lecturing to patients, use some proven ways to counter a lecture's built-in drawbacks and to increase patient participation. First, prepare patients ahead of time for what the lecture will cover. If possible, ask about their specific concerns beforehand. And when you're planning your lecture, spend some time thinking of fresh ways to make it lively and thought-provoking. If appropriate, plan to use audiovisual aids to add interest and try to incorporate some form of audience participation.

During the lecture, change the pace and tone of your talk to maintain audience interest. Invite questions and comments during as well as after the lecture. Repeat each question for those who may not have heard the original question clearly.

WATCH YOUR LANGUAGE!

Your language can improve or impair your teaching effectiveness. So be sensitive to its effect and adapt it to each patient. Follow these suggestions for making your words help your teaching efforts:

Use language appropriate to your patient's educational level or fluency with English. You're usually on safe ground if you select simple words with few syllables, make your sentences short, and use action verbs.

For clarity, break your information into large, distinct categories. You might say to the patient, "I have three important things to tell you. Number one is ...." This is a good teaching technique whether you're in the patient's room or in a lecture room.

Express complex medical and scientific concepts in layman's terms. Use analogies to make your meaning clear. Whenever possible, avoid complex clinical terms and abbreviations.

Choose specific rather than general words when giving instructions. This applies particularly to directions for the patient's medications and self-care.

Give plenty of examples and hypothetical cases to humanize your teaching.

State your most important points first and last. It's a given in teaching that the first and last points will be remembered best.

Repeat your important points. And don't be afraid to repeat them again if you feel the patient hasn't grasped them.

Teaching tools

You can use a variety of teaching tools to spur the patient's interest and to reinforce learning. These tools—whether printed pamphlets, special cassettes, or closed-circuit television programs—help familiarize the patient with a topic.

Although some hospitals prefer to develop their own teaching materials, this can be a time-consuming and expensive process. Using already existing materials is certainly more practical. When you're looking for available materials, try the inservice instructors on your unit, the hospital library, or specialists on the staff. (Of course, you can also use the many teaching aids found in this book. Keep in mind that these aids can be reproduced free of charge for distribution to patients.)

Other good sources for patient-teaching materials include the pharmaceutical and medical supply companies in your community. You can reach the sales representatives of these companies through your hospital's pharmacy department and purchasing agents.

In addition, the large national associations and foundations, such as the American Heart Association, generally have large supplies of patient-education materials written with the lay person in mind.

Many of these materials are provided free of charge; some are offered at a nominal cost.

Obviously, these prepackaged references can save you time. But of course, they in no way substitute for your own teaching; they only supplement it. Put your personal imprint on such auxiliary reference materials by marking passages that have significance for your patient and by discussing the information with him.

Some of the tools mentioned here will be available to you; some will not. But you should become familiar with the wide range of tools you can use to enhance your teaching.

• ***Printed materials.*** Books, brochures, and other printed materials are invaluable tools for presenting background information and explaining procedures. Print has the advantage of allowing the patient to read and reread the information at his convenience.

When you recommend printed materials, be sensitive to a patient's ability or inability to read and absorb information. A patient may be too embarrassed to admit he's not a skilled reader and so will pretend he can read and comprehend what you give him. If the material proves too complex or difficult, he may quickly lose the motivation to learn. Actually, the printed word tends to work best not only with the patient who reads competently, but also with the patient who has taken an active interest in his own treatment from the start.

Also determine if the patient can see well enough to read. If he has reading glasses, remind him to use them. If he doesn't have them, suggest using a magnifying glass.

The more pictures the printed materials contain, the better the patient will retain what he's learning. But take a minute to consider the best form. While actual photographs of, say, a step-by-step technique may seem to offer the most accurate illustration, remember that substituting abstract pictures, graphics, or diagrams can sometimes make a concept clearer by eliminating superfluous detail. And of course, if your patient's a child, you'll find that cartoons and pictures that use rock, sports, or movie stars will create interest and help get your message across.

• ***Audiocassette tapes.*** These tapes can be especially useful for teaching auditory and performance skills. For example, if you're teaching a parent about the care of an asthmatic child, use a tape to record normal breath sounds and wheezing sounds. The parent can then play the tape back and learn to differentiate the sounds. Also, if you're teaching a patient who's uncomfortable with printed materials, you can tape-record the steps of the procedures he's to follow. He can listen to the tape with you; then, once he understands it, he can go over it by himself.

A word of caution if you're planning to use cassette tapes or any other electrical audiovisual equipment: check your equipment beforehand to be sure you can operate it smoothly—without any mechanical hitches. With some equipment, this can take a bit of preparation and practice.

• ***Physical models.*** Anatomic models and actual equipment convey both visual and tactile information. Besides making your instruction seem more realistic than pictures, they can also reduce the patient's anxiety by familiarizing him with equipment he'll be seeing or using later.

• ***Posters and flip charts.*** Adaptable enough to be used in teaching a group of patients or a single patient at his bedside, posters and flip charts can be supported by an easel or, when necessary, propped against the back of a chair. If you're planning to use these aids repeatedly, try laminating them. This will make them easy to clean and will prevent them from becoming shabby and discolored with use.

• ***Transparencies.*** You can augment a lecture or demonstration by using an overhead projector and transparencies to project images onto a screen or wall. Transparencies can be used in a normally lighted room and thus permit you to maintain eye contact with your audience.

• ***Slides and filmstrips.*** A familiar part of lectures, demonstrations, and even individual teaching sessions, slides are displayed through a carousel projector onto a screen. The most commonly used slides are 35 mm and 2″ square. Slides can be synchronized with an audiotape when a slide-tape projector is used.

Similar to a slide and tape show, filmstrips are merely slide frames that are connected in a continuous strip. They can prove awkward and difficult to change when you want to bring your material up to date or show only a portion of your slides. For this reason, they're being used less and less.

• ***Videotapes.*** If your hospital has a centralized hookup, a videotape can be shown on the patient's own television screen. He can use earphones so other patients won't be disturbed.

Blank videotapes can also be used to record a patient while he's role-playing or practicing an unfamiliar procedure. Later, he can replay the tape and get an idea of how he's progressing.

• ***Closed-circuit television.*** Prepared teaching programs can be shown on closed-circuit television by prearrangement if your hospital has the facilities. This can provide important background teaching for a group of patients with a similar problem.

• ***Computer-assisted instruction.*** If your hospital has a computerized patient-teaching program like the ones being developed and used in many institutions, you'll have to make arrangements for your patient to have access to the computer. If he needs instruction or orientation, you'll need to provide for that, too.

Empathy: Not to be overlooked

Teaching tools are no substitute for your personal teaching. No matter how colorful, stimulating, and novel your tools may be, your patient still needs further personal orientation and follow-up. Your personal touch will add a meaning and emphasis that no aid can provide—particularly when you supply the empathy he needs.

Empathy isn't listed here as a "tool," but it is indeed a subliminal teaching device that makes your patient comfortable, builds his confidence in you, and generally fosters his readiness to learn. If you don't feel instinctively empathetic toward a patient, you can cultivate this emotion by following this approach. First, show an interest in the patient and a willingness to help him. Make an active effort to see the situation through his eyes and to imagine what he must be feeling. Keep your body relaxed and maintain eye contact. Soon enough, you'll find yourself sharing some of the patient's feelings.

PREPARING A TEACHING PLAN

Now it's time to prepare an actual teaching plan, making use of the tools and methods just explored. (See *Understanding the Components of a Teaching Plan,* pages 72 and 73.)

As you approach this task, don't think of a teaching plan as a lengthy, written document. Whatever format you use—outline, checklist, flowchart—aim to make your plan complete enough to be helpful, yet concise enough to be practical.

Preparing a teaching plan may seem like just one more thing for you to do. But this step in the teaching process can actually save you time and will certainly make your teaching more effective. Even when you can't carry out the plan to the letter—which may be the case more often than not—the organization and thought you put into the plan will pay dividends in the quality and depth of your teaching.

Tailoring the plan to fit your patient

Let's see how you'd go about preparing a teaching plan for a specific patient. Suppose your patient is Mr. Fleming, a 70-year-old retired salesman with a 9-year history of congestive heart failure. On admission he told the nurse that he "ran out of medicine." This lack of his medicine undoubtedly contributed to the episode that led to his hospitalization.

Since you discover that Mr. Fleming ran out of his medicine because of financial and transportation problems, you won't want to bother teaching him the importance of taking his medication regularly. He was doing this until he developed financial difficulties. This aspect of Mr. Fleming's problem, you realize, could be better managed by a hospital resource outside of nursing—in this case, the social services department. Knowing and using your hospital's resources will save you time and promote your patient's well-being.

Before you design a teaching plan for Mr. Fleming, you'll need to consider the goals the entire health care team has set for him. So, after investigation, you find the goals are to have Mr. Fleming learn to manage his diet, his medications, and his activities at home. Since these goals are more likely to be achieved with Mr. Fleming's cooperation and understanding than without them, you'll want to work with him from the start to make the learning goals mutual. Approach this in a casual, conversational manner, rather than in a formal interview. Determine first whether he understands that he's in the hospital because his heart isn't pumping efficiently. Then you might say, "I'd like to talk with you about taking your medications and following your diet at home. Are there some things you'd like to know more about? Have you had any problems in the past that I can help you with now?" You may find that Mr. Fleming responds well to your approach: that he's reasonable, cooperative, and willing to learn.

But you can't always count on your patient's responding positively. So for the moment, let's say Mr. Fleming is *not* eager to learn and participate in his own care. What then? There's little point in going ahead with the plan you'd normally use for his situation.

Form a contract

Establishing a contract with a noncompliant and resistant patient

UNDERSTANDING THE COMPONENTS OF A TEACHING PLAN

Whether your teaching plan is a comprehensive outline or a concise checklist, it should include a statement of your assessment findings and the patient's learning goals. What's more, it should include the activities, methods, and tools needed to accomplish these goals. Lastly, it should include the methods you'll use to evaluate the outcome of your teaching.

The chart below sets out part of a teaching plan for a diabetic patient.

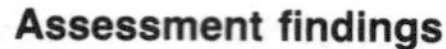

Assessment findings
Mr. Jones needs to understand the timing and action of his insulin.

Learning goals
Mr. Jones will be able to state the action, onset, peak, and duration of effect for NPH insulin.

Activities
- Present written brochures.
- Discuss content.
- Check the patient's understanding.

Teaching methods
- One-on-one discussion

Teaching tools
- Printed materials describing the timing and action of NPH insulin

Evaluation methods
- One-on-one discussion
- Written test

doesn't guarantee that effective learning and a change in attitude will take place. However, a contract *does* give the patient control over what is to be learned and allows you to make concessions—without losing sight of your overall teaching objectives.

Whether written or oral, a contract spells out each item of learning that is to be accomplished, describes your obligation as well as that of the patient, and gives a timetable. It also provides for an evaluation afterward of what learning has taken place.

How would a contract work in the case of Mr. Fleming's diet? You know he understands that salt is bad for him; yet he doesn't limit his salt intake. "I can't taste food without it," he says. Giving Mr. Fleming a lesson about the harmful effects of salt in his diet would be a waste of your time and his. You'd be going over information he already knows and chooses to ignore. But contracting with him to try other spices as salt substitutes could be the beginning of the behavioral changes you're trying to bring about.

Assessment findings
Mr. Jones needs to learn how to give himself a subcutaneous injection of insulin.

Learning goals
Mr. Jones will correctly demonstrate self-injection of insulin.

Activities
- Show Mr. Jones the videotape on drawing up and injecting insulin.
- Have him study printed materials.
- Demonstrate each step of the procedure. Provide feedback and practice time.
- Have Mr. Jones demonstrate the procedure.

Teaching methods
- Demonstration
- Practice
- One-on-one discussion

Teaching tools
- Videotape
- Printed materials
- Photographs or illustrations of key steps in the procedure
- Physical objects

Evaluation methods
- Return demonstration
- One-on-one discussion

Assessment findings
Mr. Jones reports a loss of interest in sex. He needs to learn how to cope with this and to discuss sexual concerns with his wife.

Learning goals
Mr. Jones will share his concerns about his decreased libido with his wife.

Activities
- Explore with Mr. Jones how diabetes affects his libido. If appropriate, present case studies of how other patients have dealt with the situation.
- Encourage positive responses.
- Verify that Mr. Jones has discussed sexual concerns with his wife.

Teaching methods
- One-on-one discussion
- Group discussion
- Role playing
- Case study
- Self-monitoring

Teaching tools
- Printed materials

Evaluation methods
- One-on-one discussion
- Interview

As background information, you might explain to Mr. Fleming that as he ages, the number of his taste buds decreases; this tends to make tasting more difficult. Some of the spices included in his contract—thyme, basil, paprika, marjoram, and tarragon—are strong enough to give food some taste, thus making salt unnecessary.

Determine your teaching priorities

When you're ready to outline the content of your teaching plan, you'll need to decide on your teaching priorities. Your patient may well have complex medical problems that will require considerable teaching time. You'll have to decide at the start what the patient needs to know for his protection, safety, and well-being, and what would be nice for him to know for his comfort and convenience. The reality is that what's necessary may be all you'll have time to accomplish in your teaching plan. By establishing your priorities early, you'll be better able to organize your teaching time.

FITTING A STANDARD TEACHING PLAN TO YOUR PATIENT'S NEEDS

Your institution may have developed standard teaching plans for some of the most common disorders you teach about. Here's how to adapt such a plan to meet your patient's specific learning needs.

Let's say your patient, Mrs. Porter, is a 47-year-old mother of three teenagers. She works as a housekeeper to augment her husband's salary as a school custodian.

Mrs. Porter has been hospitalized many times with chronic renal failure, caused initially by a streptococcal infection. Her disease is progressing, and the health care team feels that she'll soon require dialysis. Adjustments have been made in her diet and medications, and she needs further instruction in these areas.

In your assessment, you find Mrs. Porter depressed about her advancing disease. She agrees to be taught about diet and medication changes but has no questions. She avoids eye contact and her face seems expressionless. Her comments indicate concern about the impending dialysis.

What are Mrs. Porter's learning needs? What, if anything, will you teach her today? What tools will you use?

With the standard teaching plan as your guide, start by assessing Mrs. Porter's knowledge and skills in the areas listed. This will tell you which points to delete from

STANDARD TEACHING PLAN FOR CHRONIC RENAL FAILURE

CONTENT	TOOLS/ACTIVITIES	EVALUATION METHODS
Kidney function • Anatomy • Fluid balance • Electrolytes	• Discussion • Pamphlet #27 • Model of kidney	• Question/ answer • Discussion
Renal failure • Causes • Stages • Complications • Signs/symptoms of complications	• Discussion with MD/RN • Pamphlet #32 • Videotape #16	• Question/ answer • Discussion
Diagnostic tests • Sodium, potassium, creatinine, BUN • Radiographic studies	• Brochure #17 • Discussion	• Question/ answer
Dialysis options • Peritoneal (intermittent or continuous) dialysis • Hemodialysis	• Discussion of process (peritoneal dialysis or hemodialysis), photos 33 to 37 (peritoneal), 66 to 100 (hemodialysis) • Visit to dialysis unit with equipment preview and demonstration • Discussion of life-style changes • Identification of support services	• Return demonstration
Other treatments • Activity • Diet • Medication	• Discussion of activity • Videotape #5 • Discussion by dietitian • Pamphlet #7 • Discussion of medications by MD/RN • Medication cards for each drug	• Question/ answer • Menu selection • Medication management • Discussion

the teaching plan, which ones to include, and which ones to modify.

For example, Mrs. Porter already seems to understand renal anatomy and function, but you decide to check the extent of her knowledge and refresh her memory when you describe how dialysis works. And when you teach her about diagnostic tests, you'll explain just the ones she hasn't experienced before.

Consequently, you draw up individualized learning goals for Mrs. Porter (see below) and then determine your teaching priorities. You decide that Mrs. Porter's emotional adjustment to the progression of her disease poses a barrier to her learning at this time, but you decide to address her concerns about dialysis. Because Mrs. Porter won't be especially receptive to your teaching, you may only be able to familiarize her with the process and perhaps dispel any misconceptions. But doing this today may make future teaching sessions more productive. You decide to describe the process, using photos and diagrams, and leave some pamphlets for her to read. You also decide to discuss the life-style changes that dialysis requires and Mrs. Porter's concerns about those changes. After today's session, you'll reevaluate to see what else you may want to use from the standard teaching plan.

Mrs. Porter's learning goals: Chronic renal failure

Mrs. Porter and her family will be able to:

1. describe basic kidney functions.
2. relate personal symptoms to the process of chronic renal failure.
3. list symptoms of impending pulmonary edema and pericarditis.
4. state the reason for the necessary diagnostic tests (serum studies, urinalysis, CT scans, IVP, arteriograms, and biopsy).
5. select a form of dialysis that's compatible with her desired lifestyle.
6. state dietary and fluid restrictions as they relate to Mrs. Porter's particular stage of failure.
7. state correct administration method of medications.
8. state side effects of medications that should be reported to the doctor.

One aid you can use to determine your teaching priorities is Maslow's classic hierarchy of needs. Maslow theorized that human behavior is dominated by certain basic needs that, though interrelated, are hierarchical. The lower-level needs must be satisfied before other, higher-level needs can be met. According to Maslow, the most basic needs are physiologic. During an illness, these fundamental physiologic needs are usually in jeopardy. (See *Relating Learning Needs to Maslow's Hierarchy*.)

Applying Maslow's hierarchy to Mr. Fleming's learning needs, you'll see that teaching Mr. Fleming the proper positioning for relief of the dyspnea resulting from his congestive heart failure attends to a basic and immediate physiologic need—maintaining his supply of oxygen. Breathing is necessary for his survival and therefore comes first. Teaching Mr. Fleming about salt substitutes doesn't qualify as an immediate survival skill, but rather as a long-term need.

In short, make your teaching priorities reflect the patient's survival priorities. That way, if you don't have time on your shift to teach about salt substitutes, you can be comfortable letting the staff on the next shift handle that part of the plan. If necessary, any lessons addressing Mr. Fleming's long-term needs can even be taught when he gets home.

Most likely, Mr. Fleming isn't the only patient whose learning needs you must address. When you're spreading your teaching time among a number of patients, you'll find that ranking learning needs first by the individual patient and then across all of your patients will help you make the most effective use of your limited teaching time.

Accommodate the patient's learning strengths

Before selecting the teaching methods and tools for your plan, try the direct approach: ask the patient how he learns best. If he tells you he learns by watching and imitating, or perhaps by reading and figuring out the instructions for himself, you'll have gained a useful insight for your teaching plan. When you're ready to put this information to work, your plan stands a chance of saving time and energy for you, the patient, and other members of his health care team.

Knowing your patient's preferred learning style, you can then select complementary methods and materials. If, for example, Mr. Fleming sees himself as a visual learner, you would ideally make generous use of films, photographs, and even cartoons to illustrate the concepts you're teaching him. If he learns best by reading and figuring out the instructions and procedures for himself, you'd supply him with suitable printed materials to supplement your initial ex-

RELATING LEARNING NEEDS TO MASLOW'S HIERARCHY

If your patient has complex medical problems that require extensive teaching, you may find it difficult to put his learning needs into proper order. Maslow's hierarchy of physiologic and psychological needs can help you establish the sequence and priority of your teaching.

The diagram here shows how, in Maslow's terms, you might rank learning needs for a patient with chronic obstructive pulmonary disease. At the foundation lie the patient's basic physiologic needs, which take precedence over his need for safety and, in turn, his needs for psychological well-being and self-actualization. Your teaching should follow a similar pattern, beginning with the topics that relate to physiologic needs and progressing to teaching for higher levels of need.

SELF-ACTUALIZATION

Personal role with integration of illness

SELF-ESTEEM

Acceptance of illness-imposed role changes

Independent regulation of medication and activity

Acceptance of others' positive comments regarding care management

LOVE AND BELONGING

Maintenance of important family and social relationships

Identification with others who have similar respiratory problems

SAFETY AND SECURITY

Safe use of oxygen

Appropriate administration of medication

Recognition of complications

Management of stress

PHYSIOLOGIC NEEDS
(oxygen, liquids, food, shelter, sleep, sex)

Use of oxygen

Positioning to facilitate breathing

Breathing exercises

Activity restrictions

Dietary adjustments

planation. Remember to take a few minutes to come back to him afterward and ask if he had any problems with or questions about the material.

But don't ever feel that your patient's learning preference eliminates other tools and methods that seem suitable or valuable to you. You'll want to achieve as varied a teaching "menu" as possible to stimulate the patient's curiosity and to enable him to view a problem from more than one perspective.

TEACHING

Implementing your plan

The true challenge comes when you're ready to put your plan to work. In planning stages, all things seem possible. But when the time comes to implement your plan, you may have to take off the rose-colored glasses and become as creative as you can with the materials—and the time—you have.

Sidestepping obstacles

In short, if the wide variety of resources we've described aren't available when lesson time arrives, you'll have to get down to teaching without them. You still have the most important tool at hand: an active interchange between you and your "student."

Another major obstacle to the best-laid teaching plans is time. A staff shortage can easily sabotage your planned time for teaching. At other times, you'll have time for teaching, but your patient will be out of his room for tests. Or he'll be in too much discomfort to be receptive to your teaching. Or he'll have visitors. And so on.

As a nurse, you've learned to expect the unexpected. So circumvent the unexpected that steals your teaching time: use any moment you're with the patient to do some teaching. Don't think your planning is wasted. Your most spontaneous teaching will be better for the work that went into your plan.

Incorporating teaching into your patient care can be done in a number of ways. You can talk the patient through a new procedure, such as learning to take his own blood pressure, as you're performing that part of his care.

If the material to be taught is complicated, such as medication schedules, or comes in several parts, such as dressing changes or tracheostomy care, save time by explaining one part at a time. Do this especially when you detect a low point in the patient's attention span.

Explain what you're doing as you do it. If you're teaching Mr. Fleming how to position himself for breathing ease and comfort, encourage him to ask questions and to repeat what you've just told him. Review the procedure with him the next time you're in his room; in subsequent visits, allow him to do more and more of the task by himself. This technique, called *chaining,* allows for learning and practicing in a series of sessions.

You can also give your patient written instructions that he can refer to between teaching sessions and after his discharge. When he's on his own, these instructions can help to diminish his anxiety and to remind him of the things you stressed in your teaching. They can also serve as a hedge against backsliding that requires repeat teaching. Keep the written instructions brief and close to the information and advice you gave him in person. Refer to things you talked about—or even laughed about—in teaching sessions; this will help to refresh his memory and make the material more personal. Group the information under topical headings, which you can emphasize with large, bold letters. Add magazine pictures or your own illustrations to make the material memorable. Check your instructions carefully for accuracy, then go over them with the patient to ensure that he can read and understand what you've written. Encourage him to refer to the instructions until he's sure of the contents.

Gear your teaching to the patient's social, emotional, and cognitive needs to gain maximum benefit from his developmental capabilities (see *Relating Developmental Stages to Teaching Approaches,* pages 80 and 81).

If you identify a patient who seems unmotivated to learn and you're convinced he's resistant to your teaching, document this on his chart, explaining objectively the basis for your conclusion. Inform the doctor of the problem, and then spend your time elsewhere. Although he may be the very patient who needs your teaching and guidance the most, he's also the one who will benefit the least from your efforts. Come back to this patient later to try again—perhaps with a fresh approach. His situation and attitude can change, making him a more willing learner. However, if he remains unwilling to listen and learn, you're responsible for noting this on the chart and arranging for the required teaching to be done at discharge.

RELATING DEVELOPMENTAL STAGES TO TEACHING APPROACHES

STAGE OF DEVELOPMENT	TYPICAL BEHAVIOR DURING HOSPITALIZATION	TEACHING APPROACHES
Infant	*Under 7 months:* • Responds well to nurse • Allows parents to leave *Over 7 months:* • Anxious and unhappy • Clings to parents and cries when they leave	• Teach the parents to participate in their infant's care. • Handle the infant gently and speak in a soft, friendly tone of voice. • Use a security toy or pacifier to reduce the infant's anxiety and elicit cooperation.
Toddler	• Commonly experiences separation anxiety • May show anger by crying, shaking crib • Rejects nurse's attention • May become apathetic, crying intermittently or continuously • May reject parents and respond to nurse	• Teach the parents to participate in their child's care. • Give the child simple, direct, and honest explanations just before treatment or surgery. • Use puppets or coloring books to explain procedures. • Let the child play with equipment to reduce anxiety. • Let the child make appropriate choices, such as choosing the side of the body for an injection.
Preschooler 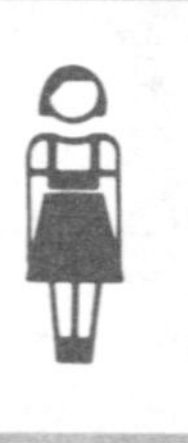	• Experiences separation anxiety; may panic or throw tantrums, especially when parents leave • Often regresses (enuresis) • Commonly shows eating and sleeping disturbances	• Teach the parents to participate in their child's care. • Use simple, neutral words to describe procedures and surgery to the child. • Encourage the child to fantasize to help plan her responses to possible situations. • Use body outlines or dolls to show anatomic sites and procedures. • Let the child handle equipment before a procedure. • Use play therapy as an emotional outlet and a way to test the child's sense of reality.
School-age child 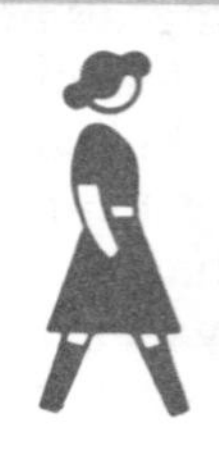	• May have insomnia, nightmares, enuresis due to anxiety about the unknown • Alternately conforms to adult standards and rebels against them	• Use body outlines and models to explain body mechanisms and procedures. • Explain logically why a procedure is necessary. • Describe the sensations to anticipate during a procedure. • Encourage the child's active participation in learning. • Praise the child for cooperating with a procedure.

STAGE OF DEVELOPMENT	TYPICAL BEHAVIOR DURING HOSPITALIZATION	TEACHING APPROACHES
Adolescent 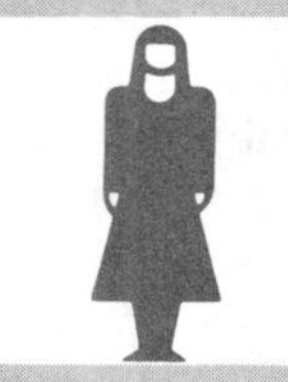	• Fluctuates in willingness to participate in care because of need for both independence and approval • Shows concern about how procedure or surgery may affect appearance	• Ask the patient if she wants her parents present during teaching sessions and procedures. • Give scientific explanations, using body diagrams, models, or videotapes. • Encourage the patient to verbalize her feelings or express them through artwork or writing. • Offer praise appropriately.
Adult 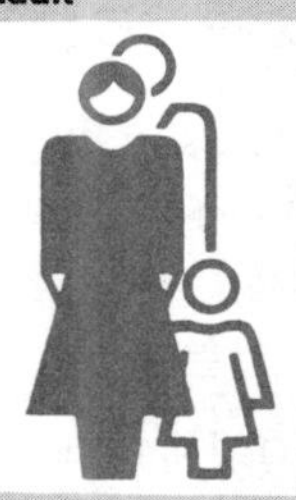	• Directs and participates in her own care • Complies with hospital regulations • Freely asks questions when she has concerns or uncertainties • Demonstrates continued interest in personal roles • Shows concern for family and economic results of hospitalization	• Negotiate learning goals with the patient. • Include family members in teaching. • Use problem-centered teaching. • Provide for immediate application of learning. • Let the patient test her own ideas, take risks, and be creative. Allow her to evaluate her actions and change her behavior. • Use the patient's past experiences as a learning resource.
Older adult 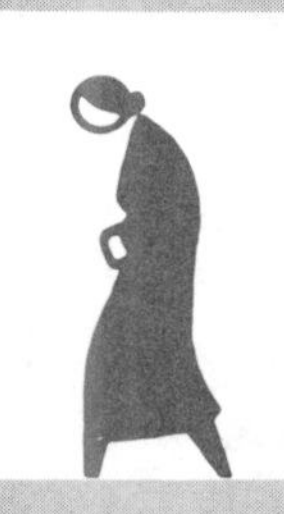	• Demonstrates anxiety over new procedures or a change in routine • Often forgets new material or ideas or takes a long time to make decisions • Maintains interest in personal matters • Asks for instructions to be repeated • Participates in care and decision making • Requires frequent rest periods	• Negotiate learning goals with the patient. • Include family members in teaching. • Schedule frequent, short teaching sessions (15 minutes maximum) at times of peak energy. Avoid holding sessions after the patient has bathed, ambulated, or taken medications that affect learning ability. • Check for memory deficit by asking for verbal feedback. • Present one idea at a time. • Use simple sentences, concrete examples, and reminders, such as calendars or pillboxes. • Speak slowly and distinctly in a conversational tone. • Use large-print materials and equipment with oversized numbers. Avoid using teaching materials printed on glossy paper.

Promoting compliance

Your best teaching will prove meaningless if your patient doesn't apply what you've taught him. If you've been working closely with him from the start, chances are greater for approaching the ideal two-way teaching-learning dynamic that promotes compliance. But now, when you're implementing your plan, you're especially anxious to have an "A" student.

Working toward compliance begins early with soliciting the patient's reaction to the teaching plan as you're formulating it. Keep his concerns in mind, and be willing to consider his criticisms of the plan or his suggestions for improvement. All of this will contribute to agreement not only on the plan, but also on what the patient's rightful participation should be.

You'd be wise to limit the number of tasks you expect of a patient at a given time. If too much is expected of him, he's in danger of doing nothing. Also, when you're attempting to reach a behavioral goal with your patient, try approaching the problem by *adding* new behaviors rather than by *phasing out* established ones.

To make the teaching process work, keep the patient as active a participant as possible. Also stress the importance of his practicing what he's learned.

Giving the right feedback

The feedback you give your patient has the potential for helping or hurting him. In giving him the information he needs to correct, improve, or continue what he's doing, you're providing concrete help. On the other hand, feedback that describes the patient himself—whether praising him as smart and cooperative or criticizing him as slow and unmotivated—isn't typically helpful and could even be harmful.

Reinforcing the gains

Success, we know, breeds success. The patient who is learning successfully is the patient likely to continue learning. The opposite is also true: lack of success can lead to discouragement and can quickly end a patient's efforts to learn.

Patient teaching, though, isn't necessarily a foregone success or failure. After all, you can influence its outcome by using reinforcement and reward. As adjuncts to your teaching, reinforcement and reward will increase the probability of your patient's learning and following his prescribed therapy.

Reinforcers vary from person to person and from situation to situation. They can be verbal or nonverbal, material or intangible.

TEACHING TIMESAVERS

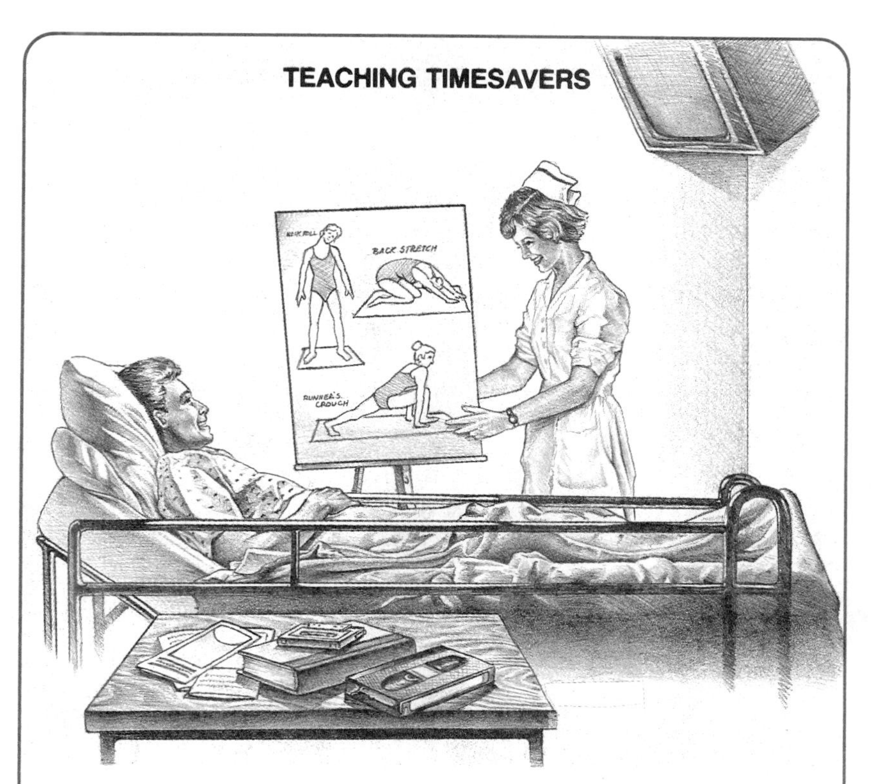

Saving your time

Consider these ways to save time in your patient teaching:

- Before you begin teaching, have the patient review written materials, audio cassettes, or videotapes to gain a basic understanding of his disorder.
- Use diagrams, charts, and other visual aids in your teaching sessions to speed comprehension.
- Rely on support staff to augment your teaching. For example, have the dietitian discuss meal plans with your patient, the respiratory technician explain spirometry, and the physical therapist teach crutch walking.
- If the patient's family will be participating in his care at home, schedule your teaching sessions during their visits.
- Teach the patient while you're providing routine nursing care. Let his questions guide your teaching.
- If you're teaching a short-stay patient and a home health nurse has been selected for him, you may want to emphasize the major points in your teaching and leave the minor points for the home health nurse.
- Document your teaching to avoid duplication of instruction.
- Document a patient's repeated resistance to teaching, and move on to teach another patient.
- Give the patient preprinted information and instructions to take home, rather than write new ones yourself.
- Once you've developed a teaching plan for a specific disorder, keep it filed for reuse or adaptation.
- Constantly evaluate your teaching to find the methods that work best for you. Then use those methods.

Saving staff time

To save time for your colleagues, suggest implementing timesaving programs that have worked in other institutions:

- Use group-teaching sessions for patients with similar teaching needs, such as diabetes, hypertension, cardiac rehabilitation, and postnatal care.
- For same-day surgery patients, add a nurse to the preadmission testing staff and make preoperative and postoperative teaching that nurse's responsibility.

They can range from a book or a piece of candy to a smile or a hug; from extra privileges to an expression of appreciation.

Some reinforcers are external, coming to the patient from you and others; some are internal, coming to the patient from within himself. The latter would include a sense of accomplishment, improved sleeping patterns, greater self-esteem, and improved body image. Sometimes, external reinforcers are added to internal ones; this happens when the patient gets comments and compliments on, for example, improving interpersonal relationships, achieving desired weight loss, or increasing his mobility.

The value of a reinforcer varies from patient to patient. For a patient who has been on an inflexible diet, a less restrictive one can become a powerful reinforcer. However, what seems like a liberalized diet to this patient could feel like a punitive one to another patient who hasn't been subject to any restrictions.

If a patient's basic physiologic needs have been met, reinforcers that help meet his needs for love, belonging, and esteem are likely to be effective.

• ***Reward the positive.*** Because reinforcement can dramatically influence a patient's behavior, you'll want to use it selectively and cautiously. Try a guideline that applies to many teaching situations: recognize what's desirable and ignore what's undesirable—unless the undesirable behavior is dangerous, disruptive, or illegal. So, if you have a demanding patient who seems to use the call bell more often than all the other patients on the floor combined, refrain from remarking about his annoying habit as much as you can. But do give him ample attention when he's not ringing the bell. He should get the idea eventually that his desirable behavior brings more rewards and attention than his undesirable behavior.

It's axiomatic that when the attention paid to undesirable behavior exceeds the attention paid to desirable behavior, the undesirable behavior is reinforced. Complaining or demanding patient behavior, noncompliance with prescribed regimens, and other negative responses can and should be overlooked. The emphasis and attention should be focused on positive responses and behaviors.

In your use of reward and reinforcement, you can't always afford to wait until a task is learned or accomplished. The patient can become discouraged along the way and stop trying. "What's the use?" he tells himself. "I'll never make it." When the goal seems particularly difficult or far away, encouragement and recognition of intermediate progress are crucial. A patient who's learning to walk with crutches or use a prosthesis needs this ongoing encouragement and reinforcement.

• ***Be specific, appropriate, and prompt.*** If you nod and say "great" or "good" to a patient, he may sense approval on your part; but you haven't succeeded in reinforcing any *specific* behavior. Make your comments specific, and indicate whether you're approving (and reinforcing) progress toward an agreed-upon teaching goal, a change in attitude, or his first attempt at a difficult task.

Use reinforcement or reward only when it's justified. Contrived enthusiasm and unfounded praise have no place in the process of reinforcement. Only genuine acknowledgment of a desired behavior will work.

Try to vary the words and change your approach from time to time. A single phrase or response repeated with unwavering regularity has virtually no power as a reinforcer. Let's say you have a patient who should be walking more. In addition to the usual encouragement, why not try a little humor or have a coffee break with him?

Give the patient his rewards and reinforcement promptly. Even a short delay can make a reward ineffective, especially if you're dealing with a young patient or a patient whose memory or time sense is impaired. The delayed reward may still be pleasing, but it won't have the same strength to influence the patient's behavior.

A FINAL WORD

While you're teaching, don't overlook the importance of the feedback you get from the patient, his family, and your colleagues. You'll find it an important stimulus to adapting, modifying, and improving your teaching.

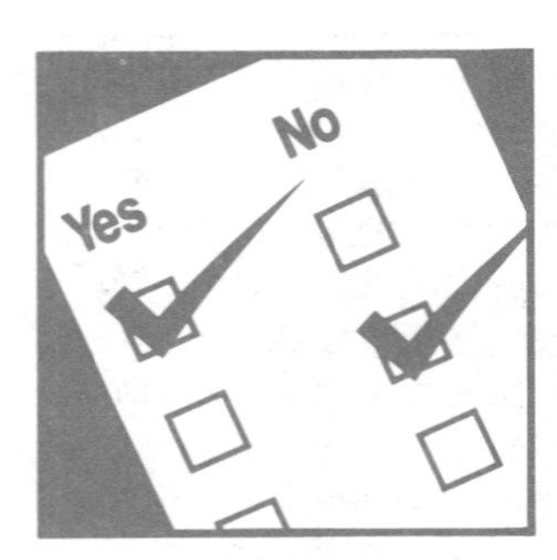

4

Evaluating your teaching

Introduction

Can the patient tolerate sitting still in a chair for 5 more minutes? Is the wound healing? Is the product doing its job?

More often than not, you ask yourself questions like these every day you're on duty. And as you answer them, you're making judgments. You're evaluating.

However, if you're like many nurses, you may not always remember to evaluate your patient teaching. Nonetheless, legislators and consumers today demand greater accountability from the health care system than ever before, and this accountability extends to patient teaching. You must demonstrate results in your teaching as surely as you do in your other responsibilities.

Evaluation is the tool you'll use to show those results. It helps you individualize your teaching and improve your skills. What's more, thorough evaluation helps you promote patient compliance and competent self-care at home.

What is evaluation?

Evaluation refers to the continuous and systematic appraisal of the patient's learning progress during and after your teaching. By comparing the results of your evaluation with the learning goals that you and the patient have agreed upon, you'll be able to judge the effectiveness of your patient teaching. Obviously, the more clearly defined and objective the learning goals, the more accurate and useful your evaluation will be.

Let's look at an example of a well-defined learning goal, one that lets you measure the patient's progress precisely: "The patient will list the five common symptoms of excessive cardiac work load." This goal gives you a clear-cut standard for evaluating the patient's success; his answer will tell you whether he knows the five symptoms or not. Accurate evaluation requires learning goals as precise as this one.

Compare this with an example of a poorly defined learning goal, which makes evaluation difficult if not impossible: "The patient will recognize unusual chest pain." This vague goal doesn't explain how the patient can recognize this pain or how different "unusual" is from "usual." How could you possibly evaluate this goal when you and the patient wouldn't be sure what it means?

As you can see, you need to clearly define your patient's goals, so that you can collect the information you need to evaluate your teaching—whether it's cognitive information, motor skills, or attitudes. With precise data and standards, you'll know how well the patient has learned, which is a good indicator of how well you've taught.

Not an exact science

Of course, evaluation isn't an exact science. Your good judgment is another important ingredient. For example, if you're evaluating a patient's skill at giving himself a subcutaneous insulin injection, you know that there isn't just one "right" way to do it. Your knowledge and experience provide the criteria for you to judge whether the patient's injection technique is safe and effective.

Perspectives on evaluation

You can evaluate your teaching from several perspectives. As a nurse, you'll of course be evaluating the learning of your individual patient. And you'll be evaluating your own skill and technique as a teacher. But you may also be asked for feedback that others can use to evaluate the overall worth of your institution's patient-education program. In some cases, you yourself may be the person who'll be evaluating that program.

Why evaluate patient teaching?

In the teaching/learning process, your ongoing evaluation constantly redirects your planning and teaching. What are some of the main advantages of this ongoing evaluation?

• ***Reinforcing desirable behavior.*** Continuous evaluation provides the basis for feedback to the patient, so you can reinforce desirable behavior.

• ***Redirecting undesirable behavior.*** Ongoing evaluation can also help you correct flaws early. For example, if your patient is contaminating his sterile eye dressing, you'll probably discover this early enough to help him learn the correct technique and speed his recovery.

• ***Measuring the patient's progress in meeting learning goals.*** Can the patient do a full dressing change or just part of it? Can he select his menu for a whole day or for just one meal? Knowing the answers to questions like these lets you determine how much progress the patient's making and how much he has yet to learn. And it addresses your foremost concern: can the patient survive on his own? Has he learned the skills and coping mechanisms he'll need to manage his condition at home?

• ***Avoiding pitfalls.*** Ongoing evaluation helps you avoid common pitfalls. For example, if a patient has trouble with tracheal suctioning in the hospital, he may not even try the procedure when he gets home. Your prompt evaluation will alert you in time to reteach him or to include additional home instruction in his discharge plan.

• ***Justifying costs.*** In a time of cost containment, evaluation can justify the time, materials, and staff used in teaching. For example, your evaluation may show that many patients benefit from physical therapy. You can use this information in a new patient's hospitalization to schedule timely, efficient use of staff.

• ***Providing necessary documentation.*** Even if you clearly and completely document your patient's learning goals and your teaching sessions, you still need to document the results. This documentation, required by the Joint Commission on Accreditation of Healthcare Organizations, serves as a legal safeguard: it provides a permanent record of the extent and success of teaching. And it could serve as your defense against charges of insufficient patient care even years later.

Clear documentation also has other advantages. For instance, it helps other members of the health care team gauge the overall worth of a patient's education program. This keeps all caregivers on the same wavelength, ensuring continuity of care and further saving time and money. Documentation can also give you "ammunition" to back up any of your requests for improving patient care or to demonstrate cost-effectiveness.

• ***Identifying effective teaching strategies.*** You may not know what you're doing right unless you check up on yourself. When you know which teaching techniques work well, you can develop a blueprint for productive teaching.

Where does evaluation begin?

Evaluation represents a kind of ongoing follow-up assessment. You should start by planning how you're going to evaluate as you plan what you're going to teach. For instance, if you plan to teach the steps of tracheostomy care, plan for each step's evaluation as you go along. Decide what data you'll need to determine if the patient's learned the step and what method you'll use to get that data.

Don't save your entire evaluation for the end of your teaching. Plan for brief, periodic evaluations throughout the teaching process. This serves a double purpose: it lets the patient immediately try out what he's learned, and it gives you immediate feedback for deciding the next step in your teaching—either reteaching the last step or moving ahead. For example, if you've just explained the types of high-cholesterol foods and their risks to a patient, let him try selecting low-cholesterol foods from a menu. This gives him a chance to try his new knowledge. And it gives you a chance to evaluate his learning, to reinforce his correct responses, and to redirect any incorrect ones. If you postpone evaluation at this point, you may later find yourself reteaching information you mistakenly assumed he'd already learned.

Immediate evaluation has another advantage. It lets you see if you're the one who needs redirection, especially if the patient doesn't seem to be making any headway. In that case, you may need to try a different tack. For example, if your patient can't correctly care for his colostomy, you may discover he felt awkward and embarrassed during your teaching session and only half-heard what you were saying. Perhaps you should try using an audiovisual teaching aid that lets the patient become familiar with the procedure in private before you rehearse it with him.

Although evaluation lets you discover which teaching strategies work best in specific situations, bear in mind that no one strategy works best for all patients in all situations.

Let your patient participate in his evaluation, just as you include him in other phases of teaching. And don't forget to give yourself time for evaluation. After all, evaluation isn't something you can sandwich between your other duties. It requires its own allotted time in your teaching schedule.

THE PROCESS

What to evaluate

Effective evaluation assesses the learner, the teacher, and the teaching strategies and media.

Evaluating the learner

Evaluate your patient against the yardstick of his learning goals: the more goals he's achieved, the better he's learned. Still, although the patient may have helped set these goals and have agreed to them, he may not be as goal-oriented as you. You must provide the motivation and direction. (See *Giving Feedback*.)

Start by letting the patient know how and when you'll evaluate his learning. Tell him the sort of questions you'll be asking and

GIVING FEEDBACK

Evaluation of patient teaching rests on a foundation of helpful feedback. The patient tells or shows you what he's learned, and you point out his successes as well as any areas needing improvement. Obviously, this exchange of information should help build the patient's confidence and improve his competence. To achieve this, though, and to avoid confronting and frustrating the patient, you'll need to adopt a positive, constructive attitude in these ways:

BE HELPFUL

Make your comments helpful, not hurtful. Share information and present alternatives, rather than dictate rules. And avoid using absolute words, such as "always" and "never."

Be sure to focus on the patient's behavior, not on his progress or personality. And discuss his *current* behavior, not his past. For instance, don't say, "That's the third time you've made this incorrect diet selection. Try it again." Instead, say something like, "Remember, carrots are high in carbohydrates. If you eat them at noon you'll have to leave them out of your evening meal, to maintain your carbohydrate restrictions."

Give the patient positive feedback first to reinforce desired behavior. Then discuss the points that he still needs to master. Otherwise, the negative comments are probably all he'll hear and remember.

BE PROMPT

Give feedback as soon as possible after you observe the patient's behavior. The longer the patient continues with an undesirable behavior, thought, or attitude, the more comfortable he'll become with it and the greater difficulty he'll have changing it.

BE SPECIFIC

Offer specific suggestions for improvement along with the rationale. If the patient understands why something needs to be done, he'll more easily remember to do it—and do it correctly. For example, you might say, "The angle at which you're holding the needle makes it go too deep. Hold the needle at a 45-degree angle instead of perpendicular to your skin."

And make sure the patient understands the feedback you've given him. If he's perfecting a technique, have him repeat it immediately, so you can check his corrections. If he's attempting something less tangible, such as changing an attitude, you might ask him to rephrase your feedback, to see if he's really listening. Also, observe other clues in his facial expressions and his offhand remarks.

BE PRACTICAL

Comment on situations that the patient can change, not ones beyond his control. For instance, if your colostomy patient has limited financial resources, don't emphasize the advantages of using more expensive disposable equipment.

BE FLEXIBLE

Move at the patient's pace, not yours. Keep in mind his needs and abilities and the amount of information he can handle. For example, instead of discussing the patient's entire drug regimen all at once, you might say, "Your medication schedule is complex. Let's talk today about just the one thing that's giving you the most trouble. We can cover the rest at our next session."

explain that you'll be asking them throughout the teaching sessions.

Structure your evaluation around the patient's successes, not around his failures. Ask him to tell you what topics *he* feels he's mastered. This lets him begin the process of self-evaluation and helps him take responsibility for his learning. For example, to evaluate the patient's grasp of your instructions about menu planning, you might say, "Let's talk about choosing foods for your diet. Why don't you tell me what you'd select for breakfast—or, for that matter, for any other meal?" Or, to determine another patient's grasp of a new procedure, you might say, "Before we look at this procedure as a whole, show me the parts of it you feel most comfortable about."

Such a learner-centered approach to evaluation lets you quickly know what the patient has learned. It also lets him start off successfully, which can go far in cushioning any future setbacks.

When your patient meets with a failure, as he undoubtedly will, discuss with him what *the two of you as a team* are going to do about it. Promoting teamwork and feedback at this early stage helps you set the stage for handling future problems and decisions. For example, suppose your patient can't apply his ostomy bag with a good seal. Without your guidance and encouragement, he might become frustrated and discouraged. With it, he might opt to use a different method of application or a different type of pouch. This way, you'll have handled a failure positively and turned it into a success.

Evaluating the teacher

While you're evaluating the patient's progress, don't forget to evaluate your own teaching skills. You can use several methods to evaluate them, but you'll probably find that getting feedback from as many sources as possible provides better data than does a solitary approach. Here are some teacher-evaluation methods that work well:

• ***Patient-family satisfaction reports.*** These short, simple questionnaires can be completed by the patient and his family at the end of a teaching session or, if necessary, at home after discharge. However, reports that go home may not be returned. (Bear in mind that patients may give only the answers they believe you want to hear when they give face-to-face feedback.)

In these reports, phrase your questions clearly and directly. Avoid negative or ambiguous questions, since they produce negative or ambiguous answers. Here are some useful questions:

□ Was the material well organized?
□ Was the presentation clear?

□ Did you find the session interesting?
□ Was the teacher's approach satisfactory?
□ Did she use a pleasant tone of voice?
□ Was the presentation paced properly or was it too fast or slow?
□ Was humor used effectively?
□ What, if anything, would improve the presentation?

Don't expect unanimous opinions and do expect some unfavorable ones. However, use the majority opinion to guide you in improving your presentation.

• ***Self-evaluation.*** As a teacher, you can teach yourself. Write down what you think are the strengths and weaknesses of your instruction. If possible, use a tape recorder to capture your teaching session. Or videotape the session, if possible, to give you an audiovisual record for later evaluation. Let your recording or written review sit for a few days; then go over it again. You'll have a fresher, more objective approach when you return to it.

Start your self-critique by asking yourself questions similar to those you asked your patient:
□ Were you comfortable with all aspects of your presentation?
□ What kind of questions did the patient and his family ask?
□ Do they point to the need for more information or a clearer presentation?
□ How well did the patient achieve his learning goals?

Accentuate the positive as you did in evaluating the patient's learning. The negative aspects can point toward improvements; don't be discouraged by them.

• ***Peer evaluation.*** Your colleagues can be some of your best teachers. Ask a nurse whose opinion you respect, or ask several nurses, to observe your teaching. If possible, show her your teaching goals and content outline. Then ask her to comment on your teaching approach and to suggest improvements.

Evaluating your teaching strategies and media

Are your teaching strategies the most effective and efficient means of instruction you can provide, given the resources available to you? To find out, you must examine how your strategies work on individual patients:
□ Are my strategies well implemented, considering the constraints of time and space?
□ Is the patient enthusiastic?
□ Am I individualizing my teaching?

If you answer "no" to most of these questions, you need to revise your teaching strategy.

To help you evaluate the media used in teaching, ask yourself these questions:

- □ Can I use media well and easily in the space I have?
- □ Does the patient have time to view the filmstrip or the videotape?
- □ Can I easily integrate media into my teaching plan?

If you answer "no" to most of these questions, the media probably aren't worthwhile and should be discarded.

Preparing for evaluation

Once you've committed yourself to evaluation, begin by focusing clearly on what you want to evaluate. Narrow your goals and set priorities for the outcomes to be measured. Otherwise, you'll waste time collecting more data than you can possibly evaluate.

Then consider what types of questions and instruments are most apt to provide you with answers. Throughout your own education, tests were probably used as the main measure of your learning. Naturally, you may want to rely on them to evaluate your patient's learning. Resist the urge. Although tests are useful in some situations, they evaluate knowledge, not behavior. To evaluate behavior, you must observe it. Watching the patient change a dressing is better than giving him a test on the steps involved.

Think about where and when to best evaluate specific types of learning. For example, you can evaluate a patient's abstinence from smoking in the hospital, but a truer evaluation may come after the patient's discharged. Similarly, some outcomes may be evaluated effectively in a single test, while others—such as techniques to lower blood pressure or cholesterol levels—will require repeated evaluation over time. Remember, too, that factors interfering with the learning process can also interfere with evaluation of learning. If you evaluate the patient when he's tired, upset, or in pain, the results may not be accurate.

THE METHODS

Gathering data

In carrying out your evaluation, you have a mix of data-gathering techniques at your disposal—and you should use a mix to provide the broadest possible view. Let's look closely at the most useful techniques.

Direct observation

In this method, often called *return demonstration,* you watch the patient demonstrate a skill or act out a simulated situation. This method works well in evaluating motor skills, such as giving an injection, changing a dressing, or bathing a newborn. It doesn't work as well in evaluating attitudinal changes since these are more difficult to observe. You might, however, become adept at reading the subtle body-language cues that signal a patient's changing attitude about doing his own ostomy irrigation or changing an amputation dressing.

You can save time with this type of evaluation by incorporating it into the patient's routine care. For instance, you can have him change his dressing while you observe for correct equipment collection, establishment of a sterile field, gloving, and handling of dressing materials using sterile techniques. You may also observe the patient's nonverbal reactions as clues to his feelings about this aspect of his care.

Besides actively involving the learner and providing for immediate feedback, observation also helps you make the patient aware of inappropriate behavior that occurs outside your teaching sessions. For example, suppose your postsurgical patient can accurately describe how to use correct body mechanics when picking up his slippers. Only by direct observation will you find out if he's applying what he has learned.

Written tests

You can use written tests before, during, and after teaching. Use them before teaching to measure what the patient already knows and what he needs to learn. Use them during teaching to measure his progress and after teaching to measure what he's learned.

Although they're useful, written tests have several disadvantages. Obviously, they work only with literate patients. They're also difficult to construct, and that's a job best left to the patient-education specialist. In addition, written tests may intimidate some patients—especially if you're using an untried test that still has flaws. Perhaps the biggest drawback is that written tests are indirect indicators of learning. As you've seen, a patient may say as you say, but not do as you say.

The redeeming aspect of written tests is that they save time. They can also measure each level of the patient's learning, from recall to synthesis.

Oral tests

Questioning the patient can evaluate his learning better than either direct observation or written tests. It lets you individualize evaluation for specific patients and situations. Like direct observation, this technique offers the advantage of allowing you to give instant feedback. Its main drawback is that it takes considerable time.

Oral tests, like written tests, demand careful preparation. (See *Creating Top-Notch Tests.*) You have to do a lot more than just ask a few pertinent questions. Here are good tips to follow for oral tests:

□ Make your questions specific to the patient's particular life situation.

□ Pose your questions tactfully so the patient won't feel he's being grilled.

□ Phrase your questions objectively to avoid giving away particular answers. (See *How to Ask Open-Ended Questions,* page 98.)

□ Try to ask hypothetical questions about how the patient will respond to situations after he's out from under your wing. For instance, you might ask, "Mr. Allen, many people who've had a heart attack feel depressed after they go home. How do you think you might handle this feeling?" Or, "Mr. Allen, if you were watching TV at home and had an uncomfortable feeling in your chest, what would you do?"

Interviews

Like oral tests, interviews are most effective when you ask sharply focused questions. Use a written outline to make your questions relate to each other, and use follow-up questions to elicit more information.

Interviews require creative listening—as important a technique as proper focusing of your questions. Try to restate each of your pa-

CREATING TOP-NOTCH TESTS

Written and oral tests are among your most valuable evaluation tools, but they're most effective when they least seem like tests. In effect, tests that seem too "testlike" may intimidate the patient and impair his performance. Here are some guidelines for making tests informative for you but less threatening for your patient.

GETTING THE INFORMATION YOU NEED

- Make tests comprehensive enough to cover all aspects of what you taught. Do not, however, focus on insignificant details.
- Emphasize understanding, interpretation, and application of the material taught—the how, why, and what questions.
- Choose questions that range from easy to hard. Test items at all levels of difficulty.
- Use questions whose answers are plausible but not obvious. Eliminate questions whose answers are suggested by other questions.
- Avoid questions with answers that follow set patterns.

REDUCING YOUR PATIENT'S ANXIETY

- Word questions as simply as possible, using language that's familiar to the patient.
- State questions clearly, so only one correct answer is possible.
- Group related questions together.
- Number the questions consecutively from beginning to end.
- Use different types of questions—multiple choice, true or false, and fill in the blanks—and give clear directions for answering each type.
- Don't ask "catch questions," which only confuse the patient.
- Give the patient plenty of time to finish the test.
- Explain how the test will be scored.
- If patient after patient seems confused by certain questions, revise these questions before you use the test again.

tient's answers. This pays dividends by assuring him that you understand his answers. It also gives him the chance to change his answers if he feels they need clarification after he hears you restate them.

Checklists

The most commonly used evaluation tool, the checklist enumerates specific characteristics or activities the patient should have mastered from the teaching session. With it, you can check off those the patient has mastered as you observe or interview him. (See *Devising Useful Checklists,* pages 100 and 101.)

Rating scales

Rating scales are practical devices for gathering evaluation data—if they're thoughtfully conceived and constructed. They have two

HOW TO ASK OPEN-ENDED QUESTIONS

Phrasing questions to get the answer you expect is natural. However, you need to resist this natural inclination in order to get accurate data for evaluation.

Review the following examples of leading and open-ended questions. Leading questions suggest a "yes" or "no" response and can limit the scope and accuracy of your evaluation. In contrast, open-ended questions encourage an accurate, complete response. You'll want to use them for collecting information for your evaluation.

LEADING QUESTIONS	OPEN-ENDED QUESTIONS
Are you physically active during the day?	What sort of activities do you perform during a typical day?
Do you have episodes of pain during the day?	What type of activity makes the pain start?
Do you eat a lot of foods that are high in cholesterol?	Tell me about your eating patterns. When do you usually eat and what sorts of foods do you usually have?
Do you shovel snow?	How often do you shovel snow in winter?
Have you quit smoking?	How much are you smoking now? When do you usually smoke?
Do you know how you got this disease?	What do you know about your disease?
Do you know how to give yourself an insulin injection?	Could you show me how you give yourself an insulin injection?

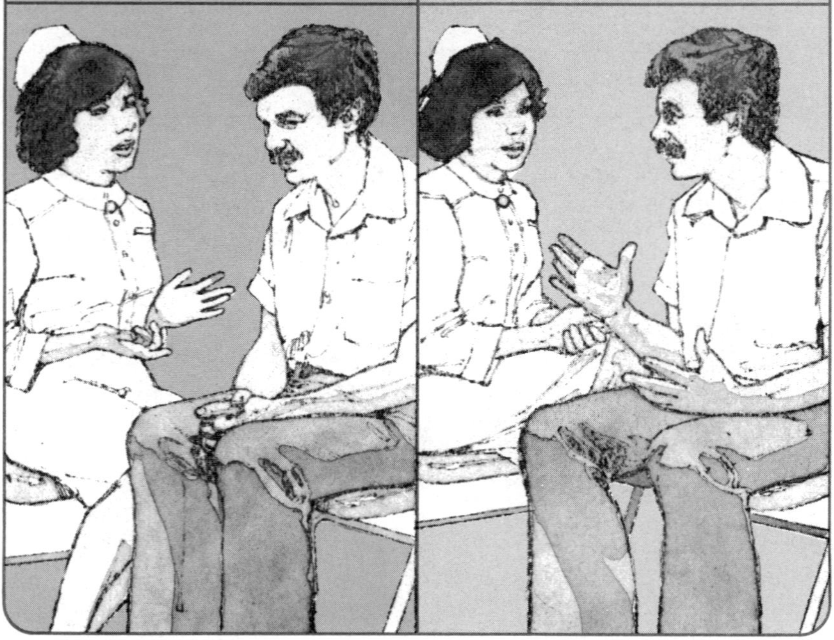

strong points: they save time and they don't require writing. You simply check the appropriate response.

Rating scales also have weaknesses. For example, you may tend to choose the middle-scale values because you don't like to use the extremes. Or you may find yourself rating patients higher or lower than is appropriate because of your feelings toward them. Be forewarned. When you use a rating scale, try not to be swayed by your biases.

Good rating scales include definitions that explain the value or weight of each of the multiple choices. They may be "anchored" by numbers (the higher the number, the higher the value) or by adjectives or adverbs (bipolar terms anchor each end of a continuum and you rate the patient's performance somewhere between the two). Commonly used bipolar terms include accurate/inaccurate, complete/incomplete, and always/never.

A rating scale may also be anchored by descriptions of patient behavior. For example, you may rate the patient who performs cardiac rehabilitation exercises by using the following descriptions for points on a continuum: needs prompting to correctly perform exercises; performs some exercises accurately with assistance or occasionally loses count and performs more or fewer exercises than recommended; consistently performs exercises independently and accurately.

Anecdotal notes

When behaviors can't be rated easily by scales or checklists, you can describe them as objectively as possible in anecdotal notes. You can later review these notes to evaluate behavior change or lack of it.

Physiologic measurements

In many cases you can evaluate teaching by the patient's physiologic status, using such measures as blood pressure level, serum cholesterol level, and activity tolerance. Obviously, changes in these measures aren't commonly seen during a brief hospitalization. Rather, they're usually the long-term results of patient education and compliance, characteristically seen on return visits or in the home. Nevertheless, researchers have demonstrated the usefulness of physiologic measures in the hospital. One study showed that short, intensive hospital teaching sessions can dramatically reduce errors in patients' self-monitoring of blood glucose levels.

DEVISING USEFUL CHECKLISTS

Checklists provide a simple, quick way of obtaining information for your evaluation. You can use them to gauge your patient's progress at various stages during your teaching.

Using checklists will give you and the patient clear evidence of what learning goals he's achieved and what goals need further work. To devise a useful checklist, follow these tips:

- Make the list concise, but wide-ranging enough to cover all aspects of the skill or activity being evaluated.
- Limit the items on the checklist to a group of related activities, such as the steps in tracheostomy care or the segments of a cardiac rehabilitation plan. Arrange the items in a logical order—sequentially, chronologically, or in order of importance.
- Identify the *essential* steps of the activities or behavior you're evaluating.
- Make the checklist items relate to the patient's learning goals and to your teaching methods.
- Use only one idea or concept in each item.
- Phrase each item succinctly and accurately.
- Test your checklist on at least two patients before adopting it permanently.
- Use the checklist along with other evaluation tools to avoid giving it undue importance.

The illustration on the right shows a sample checklist for evaluating how well a patient has learned to draw up insulin.

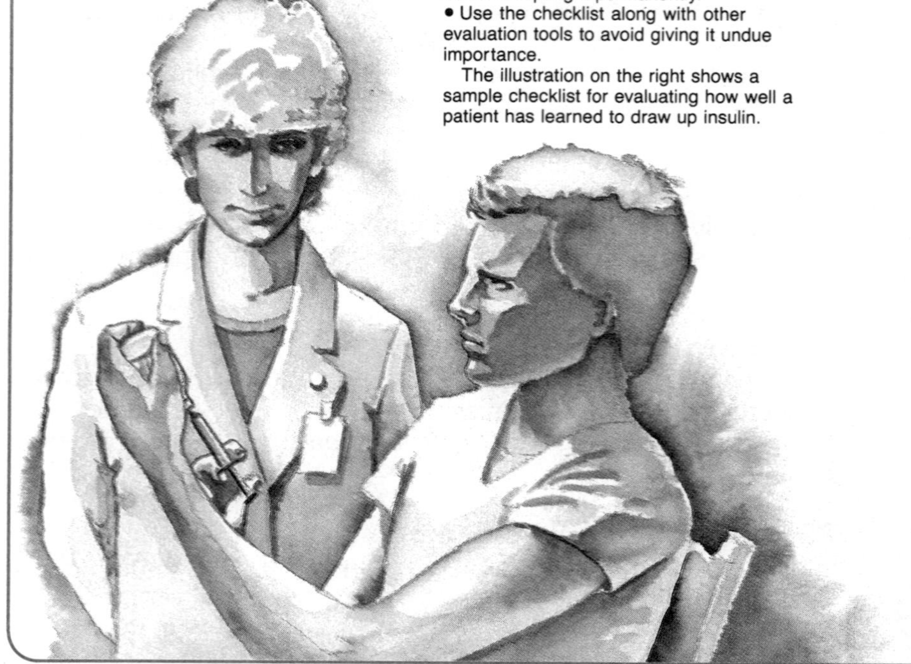

Simulation

In a simulation session, you present a typical problem for the patient to solve. For example, you might say to a diabetic patient, "Before taking a 2-week vacation to Hawaii, what plans would you make to manage your condition?"

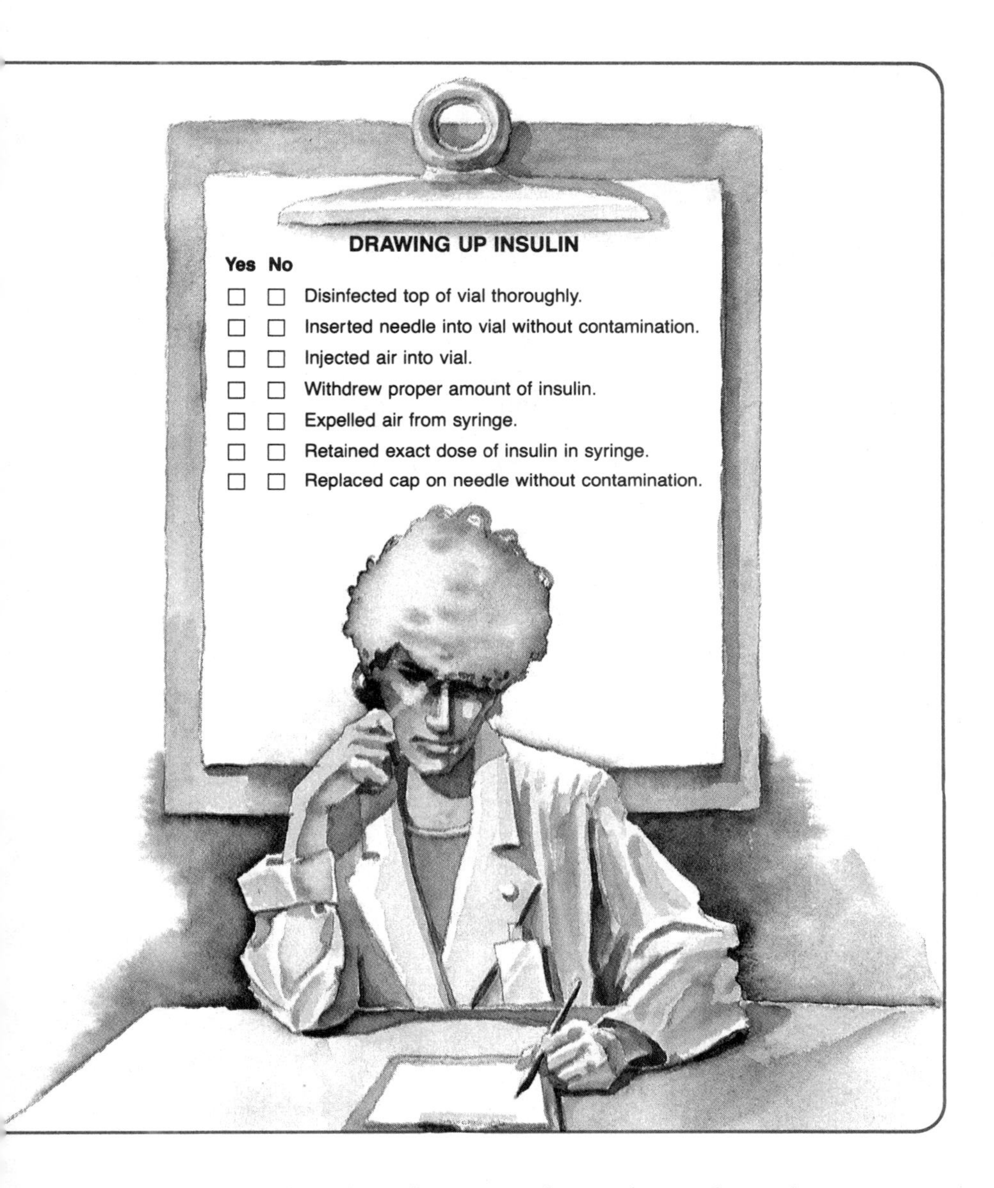

DRAWING UP INSULIN

Yes	No	
☐	☐	Disinfected top of vial thoroughly.
☐	☐	Inserted needle into vial without contamination.
☐	☐	Injected air into vial.
☐	☐	Withdrew proper amount of insulin.
☐	☐	Expelled air from syringe.
☐	☐	Retained exact dose of insulin in syringe.
☐	☐	Replaced cap on needle without contamination.

Simulation has the advantage of actively involving the patient in applying knowledge and skills to realistic situations. It's also nonthreatening. Unfortunately, simulation requires considerable time for planning and execution.

AN ONGOING ACTIVITY

Evaluation may seem like the final phase of your patient teaching, but it's not. It's something you'll be doing constantly from the moment you begin to teach.

Evaluation will help you set better learning goals for your patient at the start, determine his progress in meeting these goals, and redirect your planning and teaching as needed to achieve these goals. Evaluation will also help you recognize the skills you have that make you a good teacher and identify the ones you'll need to acquire to be an even better one.

If you strive to make evaluation a part of your patient teaching, you won't be disappointed. In fact, you'll achieve three valued goals: teaching the patient to manage his own condition, bolstering his confidence by showing him evidence of his success, and improving your teaching skills.

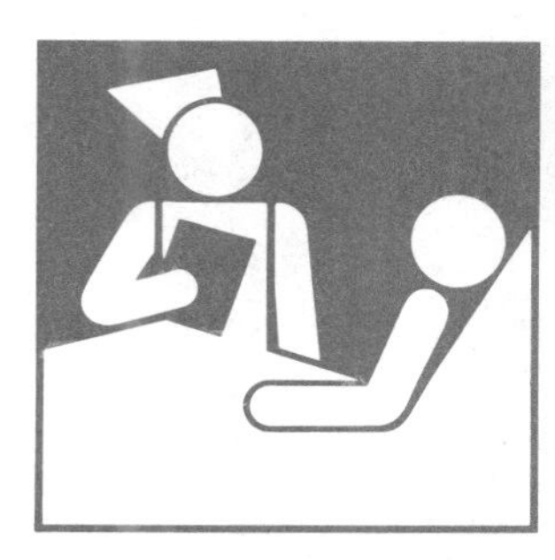

5

Core teaching topics

Introduction

All patients have questions about their disorders, about the diagnostic tests they'll undergo, and about the treatments their doctors have ordered. As a nurse, you're in the unique position to answer these questions from admission through discharge. And, in some instances, you're in a position to answer them in the patient's home. You're an invaluable provider of patient education, responsible for seeing that the patient's learning needs are met.

This chapter will provide general information that will help you teach your patient what he needs to know about his condition and the care he'll be receiving. Such knowledge will help diminish his anxiety and improve his ability to cope with hospitalization.

TEACHING UPON ADMISSION

The learning process for the patient and his family begins during the patient's admission to the hospital. Admission procedures can affect the patient positively or negatively and can set the tone for the rest of his stay.

During the admission procedure, you should introduce yourself to the patient and his family. Also introduce other members of the health care team whom they'll be seeing. Try to establish an early rapport and trust. This is essential to the therapeutic relationship and the learning process. If you appear concerned, caring, and efficient, the patient will feel less initial anxiety about being in a hospital.

Your initial teaching responsibilities include orienting the patient to his new environment, explaining safety measures, and reviewing everyday hospital routines. (See *Hospital Safety Measures* and *Hospital Routines,* page 107.) Because a hospital can seem foreign to a newly admitted patient, think of the practical things he needs to know—the location of the bathroom, where to store his belongings, how to operate the bed and the call bell, and when he's allowed to have visitors. If the patient is admitted to a double room, be sure to introduce him to his roommate.

During these early encounters with the patient, take advantage of the opportunity to do a quick, focused, preteaching assessment. How much does the patient seem to understand about his condition?

CHECKLIST

HOSPITAL SAFETY MEASURES

Use this checklist to review hospital safety measures with the patient. To prevent injuries from falls, tell him to:

- ☐ wear slippers with low heels and non-slip soles.
- ☐ avoid walking on freshly washed or waxed floors.
- ☐ keep the bed in a low position so he can get into it and out of it easily and safely. Mention that the side rails will be kept up at night.
- ☐ keep the telephone, call bell, and personal belongings, such as eyeglasses, within reach.
- ☐ use the call bell to summon help if he can't walk to the bathroom.
- ☐ use the handrails in the bathroom.

To prevent electrical or fire hazards, tell the patient to:

- ☐ plug personal appliances (such as electric shavers or hairdryers) into approved outlets only.
- ☐ restrict smoking to designated areas. Always use an ashtray. Observe *No Smoking* signs.
- ☐ stay in his room during fire alarms and drills until instructed otherwise by hospital staff.

Does he seem anxious? What's your impression of his general intelligence? His ability to speak and understand English?

TEACHING ABOUT THE DISORDER

Typically, a patient wants to know what's wrong with him and what he has to do to feel better. Before he can gain this understanding, he's going to have some questions.

"What's my condition?"

Although the doctor will usually tell the patient his diagnosis and prognosis, the responsibility for actually *explaining* what it all means most often falls to the nurse. A good place to begin is with a clear, concise definition of the patient's condition. Without overwhelming him with clinical details, try to give him some understanding of basic anatomy and physiology as they relate to his condition. Using diagrams or anatomic illustrations may be helpful. Just remember to keep these teaching tools simple and to label them with terms the patient will understand.

"What causes it?"

When discussing the cause of your patient's disorder, try to relate it to your previous explanation of anatomy and physiology. Again, keep your explanation simple.

"What can be done about it?"

Inform the patient of the expected benefits of treatment. Explain how treatment will most likely affect his symptoms. Remember, the patient has the right to determine the type and amount of treatment. You can help him decide by discussing alternative treatments.

When discussing treatment, explain how it relates to anatomy and physiology. For example, when discussing coughing and deep breathing after surgery, explain why expelling mucus from the lungs is so important.

"What can I do?"

One of your most important responsibilities is teaching the patient *his* responsibilities for managing his condition. Make sure he knows what signs and symptoms to look for to detect a relapse. If he has a chronic disorder, teach him what to expect during an exacerbation. Show him how to record the duration, location, and severity of his signs and symptoms. And tell him to call his doctor whenever they occur.

"What about home remedies?"

Well-meaning friends, family members, or acquaintances often pass on to a patient certain myths or misconceptions concerning the cause or treatment of his condition. For example, a patient may have heard that arthritis can be cured by wearing a copper bracelet over the inflamed joint. By explaining the pathophysiology of arthritis and the way in which treatments work, you should be able to dispel this myth.

"Can any groups help me?"

Give the patient a list of organizations that he can contact for financial or psychological support. If he needs further assistance, put him in touch with your social service worker. If appropriate, arrange to have a member of a support group visit him in the hospital.

CHECKLIST

HOSPITAL ROUTINES

Use this checklist when discussing hospital routines with the patient. Tell him:

- ☐ the time at which meals will be delivered to the unit.
- ☐ hospital visiting hours (including who may visit, how many visitors he may have in his room at one time, any age restrictions on visitors).
- ☐ special precautions (such as isolation procedures), if appropriate.
- ☐ scheduled times for taking vital signs and giving medications.
- ☐ information about newspapers, TV rental, telephone procedures, smoking regulations, and use of the hospital safe for storing money or valuables.
- ☐ information about his rights. Provide him with your hospital's own patient's bill of rights or the American Hospital Association's Patient's Bill of Rights.

TEACHING ABOUT TESTS

When explaining a diagnostic test to the patient, tell him exactly what will happen before, during, and after the procedure. This will promote his cooperation during the test and help ensure accurate results.

Just make sure that you understand the test yourself before you attempt to teach the patient. You'll need to have the answers to the following questions clear in your own mind first.

"What is the test?"

Refer to the test by its full name, not an abbreviation, and give a clear definition in layman's terms. For example, don't say "lumbar puncture"; say "spinal tap." Avoid acronyms that only you and other health care professionals would understand. If a test is so well-known by an acronym, however, that using its full name would be awkward—for example, "CAT" for "computed tomography"—then explain the acronym fully the first time you use it.

"What is the test's purpose?"

Explain the general purpose of the test in words the patient can understand. For example: "A complete blood count—you might hear us refer to it as a 'CBC'—shows the number and type of blood cells circulating in your bloodstream. We only have to take a small amount of blood to do this test, and it can tell us a lot of important things about your condition...."

A clear and complete explanation of the test's purpose can relieve patient anxiety, confusion, and embarrassment. If appropriate, give the patient any available literature that will amplify what you have told him. Don't rely on pamphlets alone, however, to do your job for you.

"Does anything have to be done before the test?"

Explaining pretest responsibilities—both yours and the patient's—will help ensure the patient's cooperation and the validity of the test results. For example, you would explain to a patient scheduled for a bronchoscopy that he shouldn't eat or drink after midnight before the test. (If the patient asks, explain the rationale for this: food or fluid in the stomach increases his risk of aspirating gastric contents should he vomit while under anesthesia.) Also let him know that you'll be emptying his water pitcher and calling the dietary department to have his breakfast canceled because of this restriction.

"Who'll perform the test—and where?"

Before the test, tell the patient who will be performing the test. Identify this person by name and position or title, if known. Also tell him where the test will be done. Describe the room and the equipment that will be used. This will relieve his apprehension about being taken to a part of the hospital where he's never been before.

"What will happen during the test?"

Naturally, you'll need to explain exactly how the test is conducted. First, tell the patient about how long it will take. To help explain positioning during the test, you can use sketches or have the patient practice the actual positions.

If the patient has to take a drug before the test, tell him its purpose, route of administration, and possible adverse reactions. Also explain any necessary nursing measures, such as putting up the side rails. At this time you can describe in more detail any special equipment that will be used during the test.

Think in terms of the patient's five senses when you're trying to explain the test to him. The closer you can come to giving him a clear picture of what he'll see, hear, feel, smell, and possibly even taste during the test, the less anxiety he'll experience. For example, describe what a CT scanner looks like, the clacking sound made by an X-ray machine, or the pinprick of EEG electrodes as they're attached.

Outline the patient's responsibilities during the test. If appropriate, have him practice things he'll be asked to do during the test—lying perfectly still for a CT scan, for example, or holding his breath and then exhaling fully for pulmonary function studies.

Finally, advise the patient of any adverse reactions he might experience during or after the test.

"When will results be available?"

Remember that the patient has the legal right to be informed of the test results within a reasonable amount of time. Letting him know beforehand when test results should be available can minimize his anxiety.

TEACHING ABOUT TREATMENTS

Drug therapy

Your responsibilities in teaching the patient about drug therapy will vary, depending on the setting in which you're practicing. In most cases, however, the nurse is the health care professional who sees the patient most often. So you'll probably be in the best position to teach him what he needs to know about drug therapy.

Begin by assessing the patient's understanding of his condition, his general knowledge of drug therapy, and his ability and desire to comply with the prescribed therapy.

When teaching the patient about drug therapy, be sure to cover each drug's names, purpose, appearance, dosage, and form. Also cover any special precautions or directions, adverse effects, and storage instructions. (See *Taking Medications Correctly,* pages 110 and 111.)

The drug's names

Tell the patient both the generic and brand names of each drug he'll be taking. Brand names, which tend to be shorter and catchier than generic names, are often easier for the patient to remember. Use the name that you think the patient is more likely to recognize and remember, whether it's "penicillin" (generic) or "Lasix" (brand). If the patient is being discharged with a prescription, tell him that

HOME CARE

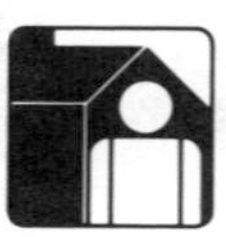

TAKING MEDICATIONS CORRECTLY

Dear Patient:

Your doctor has prescribed medication for you to help treat your condition. In order for your medication to be beneficial, however, you must take it *as prescribed*.

Safety tips

- Keep your medication in its original container or in a properly labeled prescription bottle. If you're taking more than one medication, do *not* mix them together in a pillbox.
- Store your medication in a cool, dry place or as directed by your pharmacist. *Don't* keep it in the bathroom medicine cabinet, where heat and humidity may cause it to lose its effectiveness. All containers should have childproof caps and should be kept out of the reach of children. (The top shelf of a closet is a good storage place.)
- Always take your medication in a well-lit room. Read the label to make sure you're taking the right medication. If you don't understand the directions, ask your pharmacist or doctor for clarification.
- Don't take medication whose expiration date has passed. Not only will it be ineffective, but it may be harmful. Discard the medication by flushing it down the toilet.
- If you miss a dose or several doses, ask your doctor or pharmacist for further directions (unless you were given specific instructions beforehand.)
- Refill all prescriptions promptly so you don't run out of medication when the pharmacy is closed.
- Have all prescriptions filled at the same store so that the pharmacist can keep a complete record of your medications. Inform him of any medication allergies and any nonprescription drugs you're taking.
- Don't start taking any nonprescription drugs without first checking with your pharmacist about potential interactions with other drugs you're taking. (Remember, nonprescription drugs can be harmful, too, if not taken correctly.) If you're taking a nonprescription drug, call your doctor if your condition doesn't improve after a few days.
- If you're pregnant or breastfeeding, speak to your doctor before taking any medication or home remedy. Some drugs may be harmful to the fetus.
- Your medication has been prescribed specifically for you. Do *not* share it with other members of your family or with friends; they could have a serious allergic reaction.

Administration tips

- Make a medication calendar. To do this, use a calendar with enough space to write in the names of the drugs and the times you should take them each day. Then put a check mark next to the drug when you take it.
- Set your alarm clock to go off when it's time to take your medication. Or ask a friend or relative to remind you.
- Write down the following information about each of your medications on index cards or on a chart: its name, its purpose, its appearance, directions for taking it, special cautions or side effects, and when to take it.
- Don't forget that most drugs cause side effects. Make sure you know the potential side effects that your medication can cause, especially those that must be reported to your doctor or pharmacist. If you have any questions about symptoms you're experiencing while taking your medication, call your doctor immediately.

Additional information for your prescribed medication

he may be able to buy the drug at a cheaper price if he asks for it by its generic name. Knowing this, the patient may be more likely to comply with his regimen. Tell him he'll need to talk to his doctor about generic substitutions.

The drug's purpose

The patient should know why the drug was prescribed and its desired effect. Once again, use simple language. For example, if furosemide (Lasix) is prescribed because the patient has swollen ankles, explain that the desired effect of this diuretic, or "water pill," is to help him eliminate excess fluid through urination.

The drug's appearance

Teach the patient to recognize the distinctive characteristics of his medication, such as color, size, shape, and identification code (in the case of pills). If the patient knows exactly what his medication should look like, he's less likely to get confused when taking several different drugs during the day. Once he's home by himself, his ability to recognize the right drug to take may be the final safeguard against a serious drug error.

If a generic drug is prescribed on discharge, the patient should ask the pharmacist to inform him of any difference in appearance between the new drug and a previous brand name he may be used to. When generic drugs are prescribed in the hospital, you should provide the patient with this information.

Dosage and form

Because many drugs are manufactured in various strengths, the patient must understand the dosage he's taking. This is especially important if the doctor adjusts the dosage after the patient goes home. A patient taking warfarin, for example, may be given a prescription for 5-mg tablets at discharge. Based on the results of a prothrombin time test performed a week later, he may be instructed to reduce the dose to 2.5 mg, half of a tablet.

Tell the patient how often he should take the prescribed drug. Be sure to explain whether the doses should be spaced at equal intervals over a 24-hour period or whether he can take all the doses during waking hours. Try to work out times when the patient can take his medications without changing his everyday routine. For example, taking medications just before or after meals—provided that food won't interfere with the absorption of the drug—will help the patient remember his schedule. Since patients often misinterpret prescription labels, be sure to explain what they mean in layman's language.

The patient's strict compliance with drug therapy is always desired, of course. But if a patient misses one or more doses—and patients *will* miss doses from time to time—discuss the best way to get his drug therapy back on track. If the patient misses one or more doses and is uncertain what he should do, instruct him to call his doctor or pharmacist immediately for instructions.

Tell the patient how long he can expect his drug therapy to last. This will encourage him to comply with short-term therapy for its full duration or will prepare him to accept long-term treatment. If appropriate, discuss the danger of abruptly stopping some drugs, such as cortisone or antibiotics.

Also advise the patient to inform his pharmacist, doctor, or nurse if he has any problems swallowing certain forms of a drug. Let him know that many drugs are available or can be prepared as liquids rather than as tablets or capsules.

Special precautions and instructions

Inform the patient of any special precautions he must observe—for example, not driving or using power tools when taking a drug that causes dizziness or drowsiness until he's familiar with the drug's effects. Typically, the patient will be able to drive or use power tools once he becomes accustomed to the drug.

You may have to give the patient special instructions before he starts taking his prescribed drug. For example, some drugs—such as ophthalmic, otic, and nasal preparations; sublingual and buccal tablets; respiratory inhalants; and vaginal tablets or creams—have to be administered or applied a certain way to be effective. Use diagrams, demonstrations, or practice sessions with the patient (and his family) to reinforce these special instructions.

If the patient must avoid alcohol or certain foods or drugs during therapy because of the risk of toxicity or inactivation of the therapeutic drug, explain the reasons and the possible reactions. Discuss any special procedures he must perform before he takes his prescribed drug. For example, he may need to test his urine or blood glucose level before taking insulin or to take his pulse rate before taking digoxin.

If a patient is seeing more than one doctor for various medical problems, instruct him to tell each doctor the names of all the drugs he's taking. This precaution may prevent potentially harmful interactions between prescription drugs. Also inform him that most pharmacies have patient-profile systems that keep track of a patient's prescriptions as another precaution against hazardous interactions. For this reason, advise the patient to have all his prescriptions filled at the same pharmacy.

Adverse reactions

The patient has a right to know the adverse reactions his prescribed drug might cause before he begins drug therapy. So give him a list of signs and symptoms to look for; underline the ones that he should report to his doctor immediately. Also, tell him what he can do to relieve or prevent certain adverse reactions, such as sucking on a piece of hard candy to relieve a dry mouth. As a precaution, advise the patient to always call his doctor if he's not sure about the seriousness of a sign or symptom that has developed during drug therapy.

Storage instructions

Tell the patient to store his medication in its original container, with the label clearly visible. He should keep it in a cool, dry place, out of the sun. If the medication must be refrigerated, the label will say so. Some drugs require special storage instructions—nitroglycerin, for example. If the patient is taking such a drug, tell him to ask his pharmacist about storing it. Make sure the patient knows the expiration date of his medication. Remind him that a drug whose expiration date has passed will no longer be effective and may even be unsafe. Such a drug should be discarded.

Diet therapy

Patients on a prescribed diet need to have the rationale for their diet fully explained. They may also need your help in planning acceptable meals. The dietitian will usually talk to the patient first about a new diet, but you'll probably have to clarify some points for the patient and his family.

In planning this aspect of your patient teaching, first assess the patient's current diet, eating habits, likes and dislikes, and any cultural or socioeconomic factors that have influenced his diet. Knowing what the patient usually eats and helping him see how his new diet can accommodate these preferences will promote compliance.

Most diet therapy revolves around the four basic food groups. In your teaching, you should impress on the patient the importance of following a diet that is well balanced among these food groups. Explain such dietary terms as "calories," "carbohydrates," "grains," and "protein" in relation to the foods in the patient's new diet.

Dietary instructions

Your instructions to the patient and his family should include the following information:

- ***Name of the diet.*** Refer to the patient's new diet by its proper name. If necessary, clarify the name in layman's language.
- ***Rationale and duration.*** Explain the rationale behind the patient's diet as it relates to his condition. Tell the patient how long he should stay on the diet. Generally, patients will comply most readily with short-term diets. Patients who must stay on their diets for longer periods will need more encouragement and counseling.
- ***Allowed and prohibited foods.*** Tell the patient which foods he'll be allowed to eat, keeping his preferences in mind. Of course, food restrictions must also be pointed out. Again, relate the pathophysiology of the patient's disorder to his dietary regimen. Writing out a list of allowed and prohibited foods is a good idea.
- ***Sample meal plans.*** A sample meal plan should also be put into writing and given to the patient and his family. Describe how meals should be prepared and specify the size of each portion, using common household measuring units. Define different methods of cooking, such as boiling, broiling, and frying.
- ***Important phone numbers.*** Give the patient the phone number of a dietitian or organization to call if he has any questions.

Surgery

Physically and psychologically, surgery must rank as one of the most stressful experiences a person can undergo. The stress results from what the person sees as a threat to his body, perhaps even to his life, and from the instinctive fear of pain. In preparing a patient, your goal should be to help him cope with this stress through preoperative teaching addressed to both him and his family. Studies show that patients who've been prepared through careful teaching feel less anxious about their operations, experience less pain and fewer complications postoperatively, and spend less time in the hospital than those who haven't been prepared.

You can be sure that your surgical patients will have many questions on their minds. Before surgery, patients usually want to know how long they'll have to wait before they can return to normal activities. They may even appear eager to participate in their preoperative and postoperative care. Some, however, may suddenly

PREOPERATIVE TEACHING FOR CHILDREN

Structured preoperative teaching is as essential for children as for adults. It can reduce a child's anxiety and help him cope with the stress of an operation. Here are some tips and methods you can use during your preoperative teaching for children:

- Convey concrete information using simple language. Supplement this with pictures, books, and films.
- Arrange for group tours of the surgical suite and a discussion of the surgery.
- Show pictures of doctors and nurses in surgical dress.
- Use puppets to play the parts of doctor, nurse, and patient in the operating room.
- Promote hands-on play with equipment, including stethoscopes, I.V. tubing and bottles, dressings, oxygen masks, and surgical gowns, caps, and masks. Or use life-size dolls that have incisions, dressings, I.V. lines, or casts.

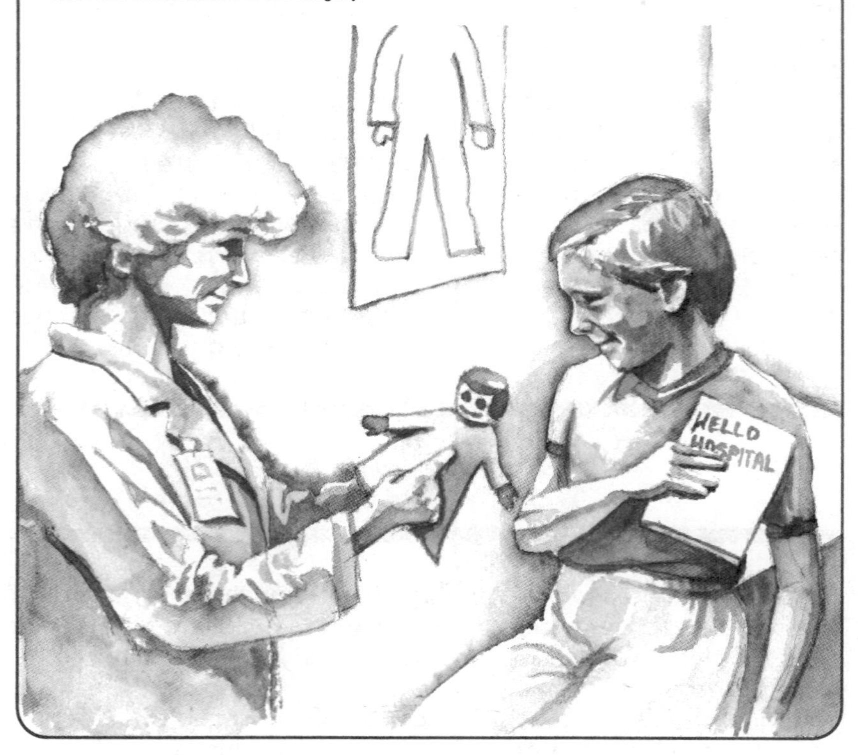

become anxious when you start to explain the surgery itself. If a patient seems uncomfortable talking about his operation and changes the subject, stop and think about how much he really needs to know. He may want to know only so much about his surgery—and no more.

With shorter hospital stays and same-day surgeries on the rise, preadmission and preoperative teaching has become more important than ever. But it must be structured to accommodate a short time period. Patterning your teaching along the following lines will help you do it better and faster.

Providing an overview

Your preoperative teaching should provide an overview of what needs to be done before, during, and after surgery to make it successful and free of complications. Your teaching should be carried out the day before surgery—even earlier, if possible—to give the patient time to practice techniques. On admission, he should be assessed to determine how much he knows about surgery in general and the operation he'll undergo in particular. As part of this assessment, you'll need to gather information about:
• past operations (type and purpose)
• the patient's understanding of the scheduled surgery
• his knowledge of preoperative routines, such as diagnostic tests and physical preparation for surgery
• his knowledge of immediate postoperative care, such as recovery room procedures and I.V. therapy
• his knowledge of postoperative exercises, such as deep breathing, coughing, and leg exercises
• his psychological readiness for surgery, fears about the proposed operation, coping mechanisms, and support systems.

Explaining preoperative tests to the patient and his family is your first teaching priority. Review the rationale for chest X-rays, a CBC, urine studies, an EKG, and other diagnostic tests. Tell the patient when and where the tests will be done. Describe any sensations he'll experience, and assure him that the test results will help determine his readiness for surgery. If the patient smokes, advise him to stop for at least 12 hours before surgery. Explain that this will decrease the risk of postoperative respiratory or circulatory complications.

Discussing preoperative routines that apply to your patient will allay some of his anxiety. For example, you may need to cover anesthesia, dietary and bowel preparation, and medication.
• ***Anesthesia.*** No matter what kind of surgery your patient is scheduled for, he'll need an anesthetic. Tell him the name of his anesthesiologist. Explain that the anesthesiologist is responsible for his care until he leaves the recovery room.

Tell the patient that his anesthesiologist will visit him before surgery and answer all of his questions. Encourage the patient to jot down any questions he has beforehand, so he doesn't forget them. If he prefers one type of anesthetic over another, advise him to discuss this with his anesthesiologist, too.

Keep in mind that your patient may have special concerns that he's reluctant to mention. For example, if he's supposed to receive a general anesthetic, he may worry that he'll suddenly awaken in the middle of the operation. Or he may be concerned about possibly never awakening at all. Try to anticipate these concerns. Assure your patient that the anesthesiologist will monitor his condition carefully throughout surgery. He'll get just the right amount of anesthetic.

- ***Diet.*** Explain the importance of a nutritious diet up to 8 hours before surgery. At that time food and fluids will be withheld. Make sure the patient understands that he can't eat or drink anything after this time. Remind the family, too.
- ***Bowel preparation.*** This procedure is usually done only if the patient is having lower abdominal surgery. Explain the procedure and rationale.
- ***Medication.*** Tell the patient what medication he'll be given before surgery and why he'll need it. Let him know the approximate time the medication will be given and describe any sensations he may feel. Explain that the side rails must be kept up and that he must stay in bed. The preoperative medication will help him relax but he won't fall asleep. Explain that the medication will make his mouth feel dry.
- ***Voiding.*** Instruct the patient to void immediately before preoperative medications are given. For some surgical procedures, the patient will need to be catheterized before the operation. Explain the procedure to the patient.
- ***Skin preparation.*** Preoperative skin preparation and hair removal may have a negative effect on the patient's body image. Carefully explain the rationale—to prevent surgical wound infection by cleansing the skin of microorganisms, some of which are found in body hair.
- ***I.V. therapy.*** Discuss I.V. therapy in terms of the site and technique to be used. Tell the patient if an I.V. will be started before he goes to surgery or after he gets to the operating room. Explain that fluids and nutrients, given during surgery, help prevent postoperative complications.
- ***Clothing.*** Instruct your patient to remove jewelry, eyeglasses or contact lenses, prostheses (including dentures), wigs, makeup, and nail polish. Explain that you can tape a plain wedding band to his finger. Give the patient a gown and surgical cap to put on. Assure him that his privacy will be respected with proper draping.
- ***Family waiting area.*** Show the patient's family where they can wait during the operation. If they want to visit the patient preoperatively, tell them to arrive 2 hours before the surgery.
- ***Operating room.*** Transfer time, procedures, and techniques also need to be explained to the patient. Once again, describe sensations

the patient will experience. Warn him that he may have to wait a short time in the holding area before he's taken into the operating room. Explain that the doctors and nurses will be in surgical dress and that even though they'll be observing him closely, they probably won't talk to him. Tell him that this will allow the medication to take effect.

Advise the patient that he'll be taken to the operating room on a stretcher and transferred from the stretcher to the operating room table. For his own safety, he'll be strapped securely to the table. The operating room nurses will check his vital signs frequently.

Warn the patient that the operating room may feel cool. Electrodes may be put on his chest to monitor his heart rate during surgery. Describe the drowsy, floating sensation he'll feel as the anesthetic is administered. Tell him it's important that he relax at this time.

- ***Recovery room.*** To allay the patient's anxiety, briefly describe the sensations he'll experience after the anesthetic wears off. Let him know how long he'll be in the recovery room. Tell him that the recovery room nurse will call his name, then ask him to answer some questions and follow some simple commands, such as wiggling his toes. Tell him that he may feel pain at the surgical site, but the nurses will try to minimize it.

Describe the oxygen delivery device, such as a nasal cannula, that he'll need after surgery. Explain that once he's recovered from the anesthesia, he'll be taken back to his room. Tell him that he'll be able to see his family, but that he'll probably feel drowsy and may want to nap for the rest of the day. Make sure he knows that you'll be taking his blood pressure and pulse frequently as a routine precaution. That way he won't become alarmed and think something's wrong.

Controlling pain

A surgical patient is usually anxious about how much pain he'll feel after his operation. You can help reduce his anxiety by advising him of pain-control measures that you'll be using. You can also teach him when to ask for pain medication and how to use certain pain-control measures on his own.

Briefly, point out to him that pain usually occurs after surgery because of stimulation of nerve endings in the skin, as well as from tissue swelling and organ manipulation. Postoperative pain typically lasts 24 to 48 hours but may last longer with extensive surgery.

Now discuss specific measures that can be used to prevent or relieve incisional pain. (See *How to Reduce Incisional Pain,* page 120.)

Explain that the doctor will order pain medication to be given every 3 to 4 hours, if needed. Instruct the patient to describe his

HOME CARE

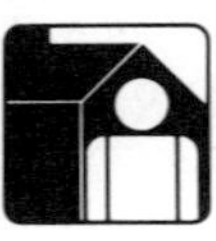

HOW TO REDUCE INCISIONAL PAIN

Dear Patient:

To help reduce pain when you move, cough, or breathe deeply, you'll need to observe precautions and, perhaps, learn how to splint your incision.

Observing precautions

- Use the bed's side rails for support when you move and turn.
- Move slowly and steadily. Don't move quickly or jerkily.
- Whenever possible, wait to move until *after* your pain medication has taken effect.
- Frequently move those parts of your body that weren't affected by surgery to prevent them from becoming stiff and sore.
- If you have difficulty moving by yourself, ask the nurse or a family member to help.

Splinting your incision

If you've had chest or abdominal surgery, splinting the incision may help reduce pain when you cough or move.

You can do this by placing one hand above and the other hand below your incision, then pressing gently and breathing normally when you move. (The patient shown in the illustration at the top of the next column has a chest wall incision.)

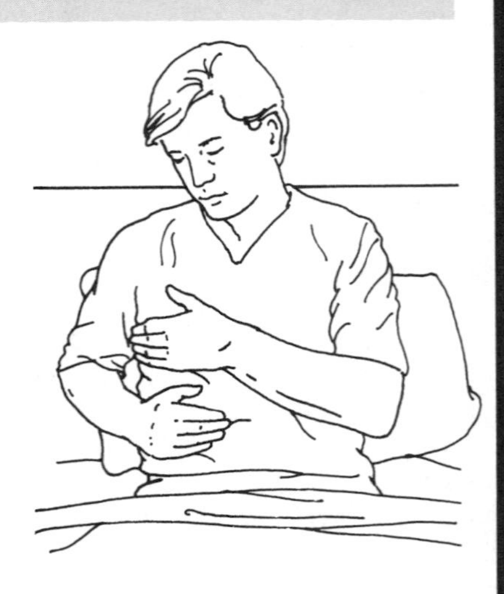

Or you can place a small pillow over the incision. Hold it in place with your hands and arms, as shown below. Press gently, breathe normally, and move to a sitting or standing position.

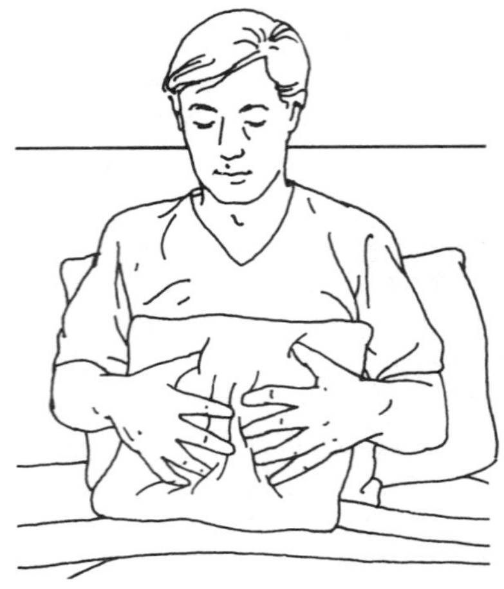

pain in terms of its quality, severity, and location. Encourage him to let you know as soon as he feels any pain instead of waiting until it becomes intense. Pain can be controlled better if it's managed early. Discuss how the medication will be administered—whether by injection or orally (once the patient resumes eating, usually 48 hours postoperatively). Identify the type of medication to be given (for example, a narcotic or an analgesic), and explain how it works to control pain.

Tell the patient which nursing measures you'll use to relieve pain and promote comfort, such as positioning, diversional activities, and splinting.

Preventing complications

The best way to prevent postoperative complications is by teaching the patient *preoperatively* the techniques of early mobility and ambulation, coughing and deep breathing, use of an incentive spirometer, and leg exercises.

Tell the patient that early mobility and ambulation increase the rate and depth of breathing, preventing atelectasis and hypostatic pneumonia. With increased cerebral oxygenation, he'll feel more alert and more optimistic about his recovery. Circulation will improve as a result of early mobility, promoting renal perfusion and urine production. Thrombophlebitis from venous stasis may also be prevented.

Early ambulation quickens peristalsis, which usually slows to a halt during surgery from the effects of the anesthetic. Postoperative constipation and abdominal distention can thus be diminished. Finally, early ambulation increases metabolism and prevents loss of muscle tone.

Coughing and deep breathing prevent atelectasis after surgery. Explain to the patient that to deep-breathe correctly, he must use his diaphragm and abdominal muscles and not just his chest muscles. Tell him to practice two or three times a day before surgery, if possible. Maneuvers should be done 30 minutes after pain medication is administered and should be repeated every 1 to 2 hours. (See *How to Cough and Deep-Breathe,* pages 122 and 123.)

Incentive spirometers encourage the patient to deep-breathe and provide feedback on how well he's doing. (See *Learning about Spirometers,* page 124.)

Simple leg exercises—such as alternately contracting and relaxing the calf and thigh muscles—will prevent venous pooling.

HOME CARE

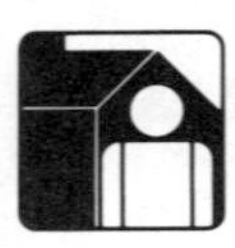

HOW TO COUGH AND DEEP-BREATHE

Dear Patient:

Coughing and deep-breathing exercises will speed your recovery and reduce the risk of respiratory complications.

How to cough

Practice coughing exercises before surgery. After it, you'll need to do them at least every 2 hours to help keep your lungs free of secretions.

1

If your condition permits, sit on the edge of your bed. Ask for a stool if your feet don't touch the floor. Lean slightly forward.

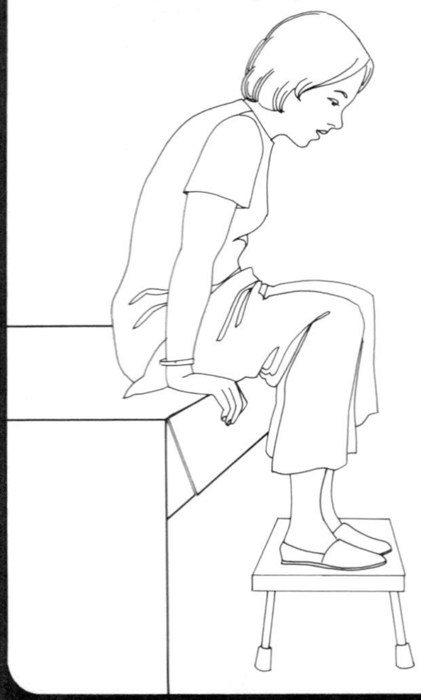

(After surgery, you can perform this exercise while lying in a comfortable position instead of sitting on the edge of the bed.) Bend your legs to support your abdominal muscles.

If you're scheduled for chest or abdominal surgery, splint your "incision" before you cough.

2

To help stimulate your cough reflex, take a slow, deep breath. Breathe in through your nose and concentrate on fully expanding your chest. Breathe out through your mouth, and concentrate on feeling your chest sink downward and inward. Then take a second breath in the same manner.

3

Now take a third deep breath, but this time hold your breath. Then cough two or three times in a row (once is not enough). This will clear your breathing passages. As you cough, concentrate on feeling your diaphragm force out all the air in your chest. Then take three to five normal breaths, exhale slowly, and relax.

Repeat this exercise at least once. Don't worry about your stitches splitting. They're very strong.

How to deep-breathe

Performing deep-breathing exercises several times an hour helps keep your lungs fully expanded.

To deep-breathe correctly, you must use your diaphragm and abdominal muscles—not just your chest muscles. This exercise teaches you how. Practice it two or three times a day before surgery, as follows:

1

Lie on your back in a comfortable position. Place one hand on your chest and the other over your upper abdomen, as shown in the illustration below. Bend your legs slightly and relax.

Exhale normally. Then close your mouth and inhale deeply through your nose. Concentrate on feeling your abdomen rise. Don't expand your chest. If the hand on your abdomen rises as you inhale, you're breathing correctly.

Hold your breath and slowly count to five.

2

Purse your lips as though about to whistle, then exhale completely through your mouth. Don't let your cheeks puff out. Using your abdominal muscles, squeeze all the air out. Your ribs should sink downward and inward. Try not to take intermittent shallow breaths during this full exhalation.

3

Rest several seconds, then repeat the exercise until you've done it 5 to 10 times.

Note: You can also do this exercise while lying on your side, sitting, or standing, or as you're turning in bed.

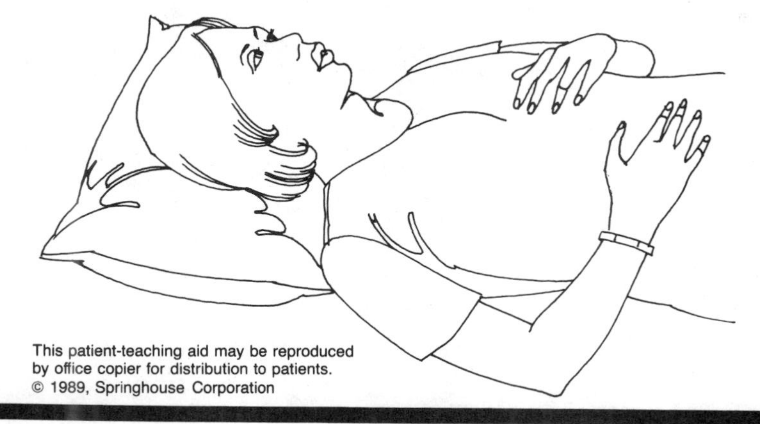

LEARNING ABOUT SPIROMETERS

Preoperatively, your patient may understand why deep-breathing exercises are important. But after surgery, when he's weak, sedated, or in pain, he may need some encouragement to do them regularly. Incentive spirometry, which provides instant feedback, may give him the encouragement he needs.

Before you teach your patient how to use incentive spirometers, compare and review the two different types. Even though all spirometers are designed to encourage slow, sustained maximal inspiration, they can be divided into *flow incentive* and *volume incentive* types. A flow incentive spirometer measures the patient's inspiratory effort (flow rate) in cubic centimeters per second (cc/second). A volume incentive spirometer goes one step further. From the patient's flow rate, it calculates the *volume* of air the patient inhales. Because of this extra step, many volume incentive spirometers are larger, more complicated, and more expensive than flow incentive spirometers.

If the patient is to use a volume incentive spirometer, the doctor or respiratory therapist will order a *goal volume* (in cubic centimeters) for the patient to reach. This will be the amount of air the patient should inspire when he takes a deep breath.

With one type of volume incentive spirometer, the goal volume will be displayed on the machine. As the patient inhales, the volume of air he's taking into his lungs will also be shown, climbing a scale until he reaches or surpasses the goal volume. This will not only help him fully expand his lungs, but will also provide immediate feedback as to how well he's doing.

The patient will usually do this exercise five times each day. Between exercises he should rest. Each morning he should reset the goal-volume-achieved display so he can try to do even better.

With another type of volume incentive spirometer, smaller and easier to use, the patient inhales slowly and deeply as a piston inside a cylinder rises to meet the preset volume. The number of exercises the patient should do each day remains the same.

Flow incentive spirometers have no preset volume. These spirometers usually have three cylinders, each containing a colored ball. As the patient inhales, the balls rise, one at a time. The patient's flow rate is measured in cc/second. For example, when the first ball rises, the flow rate may be 600 cc/second; the second ball, 900 cc/second; and the third ball, 1,200 cc/second. The number of exercises the patient should do each day is the same as with volume incentive spirometers.

Which type of spirometer is better for your patient?
That depends. For low-risk patients, a flow incentive spirometer would probably be better. Lightweight and durable, it can be left at the bedside for the patient to use even when you're not there to supervise.

But if your patient is at high risk for developing atelectasis, a volume incentive spirometer may be preferred. Because it measures lung inflation more precisely, this type of spirometer helps you determine whether your patient is inhaling adequately.

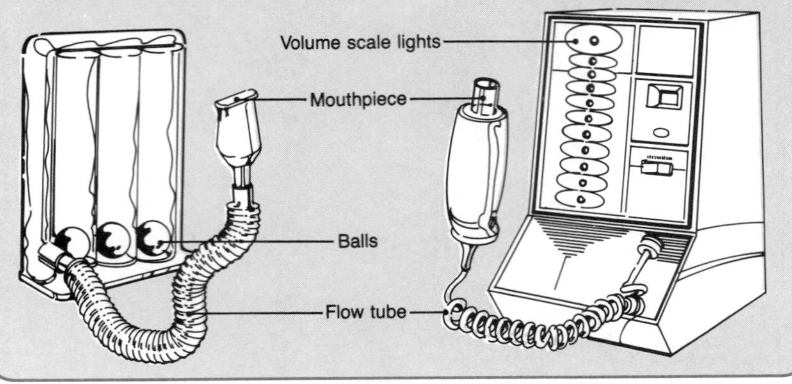

DISCHARGE TEACHING

Effective discharge teaching begins immediately after admission and takes into account the initial assessment of the patient's understanding of his condition, surgery or other treatment, and postoperative care. Discharge teaching must include the patient's family or other caregivers to ensure that he receives proper home care.

Home care requirements

Begin determining the patient's home care requirements by finding out how much walking he'll have to do at home. What's the floor plan of his house or apartment, for example? Will he need to climb stairs? Let the patient know how soon he should be able to drive a car or return to work.

If the patient has had surgery, inform him or a family member to observe the incision daily for warmth, redness, and swelling. Unless he's been given other instructions, explain that he should use clean water to wash the incision. Tell him to keep the incision clean and dry and to discard dressings in a plastic trash bag. Teach proper hand-washing technique. Discuss when the patient can bathe, and specify whether he should take a shower or bath.

Discuss the doctor's recommendations concerning activity and exercise level, relating them to the patient's everyday routine. After surgery, patients are often advised not to lift a heavy weight, such as a basket of laundry. Make sure the patient and his family understand such restrictions.

Review dietary restrictions and meal plans. Recommend a good diet book, and refer the patient to a dietitian for further information.

If the patient needs to rent or purchase special equipment, such as a hospital bed or walker, give him a list of suppliers in the area.

Finally, teach the patient and his family about emergency care procedures. Provide written instructions on reportable signs and symptoms, such as bleeding or discharge from an incision or acute incisional pain. Advise the patient to keep his follow-up medical appointments and to call the doctor with any questions.

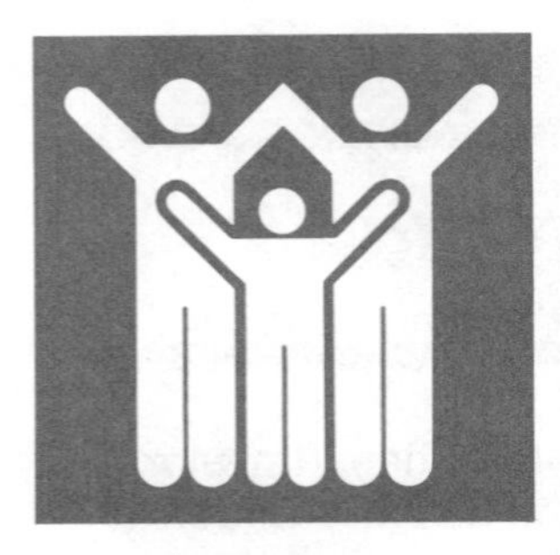

6 Health promotion

Introduction

Research continues to provide mounting evidence that poor health practices contribute to a wide range of illnesses, a shortened life span, and spiraling health care costs. In contrast, good health practices have just the opposite effect: fewer illnesses, a longer life span, and lower health care costs. What's more, good health practices can benefit most people no matter at what stage of life they're begun. Of course, the earlier they're begun, the less they have to overcome. But, fortunately, later is better than never.

That's an important idea to remember, because poor health practices persist despite overwhelming evidence linking them to debilitating and even fatal illness. For example, we've known for over 20 years that smoking causes cancer and other serious illnesses. And we know that year after year far more people die from smoking-related lung disease than from car, plane, and train accidents combined. Despite this knowledge, millions still smoke. However, on the positive side, even long-term smokers who quit may experience reversal of adverse cardiovascular and respiratory effects.

What is health promotion?

Quite simply, it's teaching good health practices and finding ways to help people correct their poor health practices. It's something that you'll do in a variety of settings—from your clinic, hospital, or patient's home to a community meeting, church social, or backyard barbecue.

But what specifically should you teach? One good place to start is with the U.S. Surgeon General's 1976 report, which outlines major health problems. This report divides the life cycle into five stages—infancy, childhood, adolescence, adulthood, and old age—and sets goals to promote health and reduce mortality for each stage.

You can use the Surgeon General's goals to direct your teaching. For example, to promote health in *infancy*, you'll need to stress the importance of prenatal care to help prevent low birth weight and certain birth defects. By educating parents about childbirth alternatives, you can also improve the chances of a safe delivery. Other topics that you'll need to cover include infant safety and nutrition.

Because accidents account for almost half of all fatalities in *childhood*, you'll need to emphasize such safety measures as consistent use of seat belts and precautions to prevent burns and poisoning. Your teaching must also stress nutrition to enhance growth and development, immunization against infectious diseases, and proper dental care.

To promote health in *adolescence*, you'll need to teach how to prevent motor vehicle accidents, drug and alcohol abuse, and suicide. You'll also need to provide information about contraception and proper care during pregnancy.

Some adolescent problems carry over into *adulthood*. However, the leading causes of death in this age-group are heart disease, cancer, and cerebrovascular accident (CVA). To promote health in adulthood, you'll need to cover such topics as how to quit smoking and how to perform self-examination of the breasts or testes.

To promote health in *old age*, you'll need to teach how to maintain independence through proper nutrition and exercise. You may also need to provide advice on coping with the effects of aging, such as hearing loss, and on preventing life-threatening infection.

HEALTH IN INFANCY

Providing prenatal instruction

How a woman cares for herself during pregnancy directly affects the health of her unborn infant. Two factors especially can jeopardize the infant's health: low birth weight (LBW) and birth defects. Any infant weighing less than 5½ lb (2.5 kg) at birth falls into this LBW category. Such infants are more likely to develop complications and less likely to survive them.

To promote the birth of a healthy infant, your teaching must stress the importance of early and ongoing prenatal care. Encourage a pregnant woman to schedule her first prenatal visit during the first trimester. After that, she should keep her appointments for follow-up visits, which are usually monthly through the 28th week of gestation, every 2 weeks between weeks 29 and 36, and then once a week until delivery.

During the first prenatal visit, you'll help obtain a thorough patient history and physical examination, including laboratory tests. When taking the history, be sure to ask about any genetic disorders in the patient's family and about any previous pregnancies. Next, obtain a baseline blood pressure reading, and measure the patient's height and weight. Explain laboratory tests, which may include VDRL, Pap smear, hemoglobin/hematocrit, urinalysis for glucose and protein, Rh factor and blood group, and rubella titer.

During the patient's subsequent prenatal visits, check her blood pressure and weight, and collect a urine specimen for analysis. Explain that the doctor will assess fetal well-being—usually by palpation and auscultation—and may recommend an amniocentesis, if indicated. Focus most of your teaching efforts on prenatal nutrition and exercise and the adverse effects of cigarette smoking, alcohol, caffeine, and drugs on the fetus. Also, teach the patient how to avoid exposure to certain infectious and toxic agents associated with birth defects. If the hospital in your area has childbirth education classes, suggest that the patient and her coach attend them to prepare for labor and delivery and to learn about infant care.

Ensuring nutrition for two

Because the fetus relies on the mother for nourishment, poor nutrition during pregnancy can adversely affect intrauterine growth and development. Obstetricians once limited weight gain during pregnancy in the belief that smaller babies ensured easier—and thus, safer—deliveries. But now most recommend a weight gain of 25 to 30 lb during pregnancy. This weight gain should not represent "empty calories" but a diet that's geared to the nutritional needs of the mother and her unborn child.

• ***Caloric intake.*** Advise the pregnant woman to increase her caloric intake by about 300 calories per day, depending on how rapidly she's gaining weight. Generally, she should be eating no fewer than 1,800 calories per day.

Make sure she understands the importance of selecting nutritious foods—and not "junk food"—to bolster her caloric intake. Also explain how the body metabolizes protein for energy if caloric intake is inadequate. This, in turn, robs the mother and fetus of protein for tissue growth.

• ***Protein requirements.*** Pregnancy increases a woman's protein requirement from 44 g of protein per day to 74 g per day. This extra protein supports increased maternal blood volume and tissue growth in the uterus, breasts, placenta, and fetus.

Because the American diet is high in protein, most expectant mothers are in no danger of protein deficiency. However, encourage the pregnant woman to eat high-quality protein of animal origin, such as plenty of meat, milk, eggs, cheese, poultry, and fish. If she's a vegetarian, teach her about protein alternatives, such as legumes, nuts, and meat analogues (soy).

• ***Vitamin and mineral supplements.*** Teach the pregnant woman that vitamins and minerals are intended to supplement, not replace,

a well-balanced diet. Tell her to take prenatal vitamins and possibly an iron supplement, as directed by her obstetrician or nurse-midwife.
• ***Salt restrictions.*** Instruct her to limit her use of salt and to avoid high-sodium foods to prevent fluid retention.
• ***Fiber.*** To avoid constipation and hemorrhoids during pregnancy, teach the pregnant woman to add fiber—such as whole grain breads, high-fiber cereals, legumes, and fruits and vegetables—to her diet.
• ***Fluid requirements.*** Help her stay well hydrated during pregnancy by recommending that she drink at least 8 glasses of fluid each day, including 4 to 6 glasses of water.

Promoting fitness

The benefits of prenatal exercise are many. For example, it can reduce or eliminate back pain, stress, depression, fatigue, constipation, and calf cramps. However, warn the pregnant woman not to overdo it.

Instruct her to consult her doctor about an exercise program, especially if she is accustomed to a sedentary life-style; is obese or markedly underweight; has hypertension, anemia or other blood disorders, thyroid disease, diabetes, cardiac dysrhythmia or palpitations; or has a history of precipitous labor, intrauterine growth retardation, bleeding during pregnancy, or breech presentation in the last trimester. Under no circumstances should she exercise if she has ruptured membranes, premature labor, multiple gestation, an incompetent cervix, placenta previa, cardiac disease, or a history of three or more spontaneous abortions.

Warning about alcohol, caffeine, and drugs

Warn the expectant mother that alcohol consumption during pregnancy increases the risk of having an LBW infant or one with birth defects and/or mental retardation. Explain that researchers still don't know how many drinks per day during pregnancy is safe.

The stimulant caffeine can cause birth defects in animals when ingested in large quantities. While a link between caffeine and birth defects in humans hasn't been proven, encourage the pregnant woman to limit her intake of coffee, tea, soda, and chocolate.

Since many drugs cross the placenta to the fetus, also tell her not to take *any* medications, including aspirin, without her doctor's permission.

Discouraging smoking

One of the Surgeon General's warnings on cigarette packs reads "Smoking causes lung cancer, heart disease, and emphysema, and

HOME CARE

EATING RIGHT: HELPING YOU HAVE A HEALTHY BABY

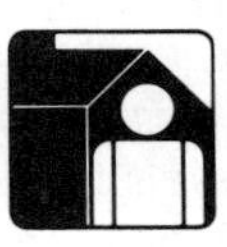

Dear Patient:

What you eat when you're pregnant affects both you and your unborn baby. That's why it's important to eat the right foods from the moment you learn you're pregnant. Just follow these nutrition tips.

Protein and calories

You need almost one and a half times the amount of protein now that you're pregnant. Choose from good protein sources, such as lean meat, milk, eggs, cheese, poultry, and fish.

You also need at least 1,800 calories per day and perhaps a lot more, depending on your height and weight. Ask your doctor or nurse-midwife for calorie requirements for a person your size. Generally, you should consume about 300 calories more per day than you usually do. When adding calories, choose from the following four groups: milk group (cheese, ice cream, and other milk products), meat group (meat, fish, poultry, eggs, cheese, or legumes), fruit and vegetable group (dark green or yellow vegetables, citrus fruit, or tomatoes), and bread and cereal group (whole grain bread or cereal, rice, or pasta).

Vitamins and minerals

Use only those supplements prescribed by your doctor or nurse-midwife. Don't take over-the-counter megavitamins since they might have an ill effect on your unborn baby.

Fiber and fluids

You need an adequate amount of fiber in your diet to help prevent constipation, which can cause hemorrhoids. Include whole grain breads and cereals, legumes, fruits, and vegetables. Add fiber to your diet gradually to avoid the possibility of diarrhea.

Remember to drink plenty of fluids, especially during the summer months and before, during, and after exercise. Unless your doctor directs otherwise, drink 4 to 6 glasses of water plus another 2 to 4 glasses of fluid each day.

Cautious consumption

Many health professionals advise steering clear or reducing consumption of "junk foods," dietetic products, caffeinated beverages like coffee and regular colas, and alcohol during pregnancy. Check with your doctor or nurse-midwife for instructions.

may complicate pregnancy." And with good reason. Infants born to women who smoke weigh an average of 6 oz (170 g) less than infants born to women who don't smoke. Nicotine constricts blood vessels, which in turn decreases the oxygen level in the blood that reaches the fetus. Besides lowering an infant's birth weight, smoking during pregnancy increases the chance of spontaneous abortion or stillbirth. Pregnant women smoking one or more packs of cigarettes a day have a 50% greater risk of infant mortality.

Obviously, the less a pregnant woman smokes, the better. Many women are highly motivated to stop smoking, or at least to curb this habit, once they learn they're pregnant. Take this opportunity to encourage a woman to stop smoking for good.

Advising about rubella: Risk factor for birth defects

Exposure to rubella, or German measles, during pregnancy—especially in the first trimester—increases the risk of congenital abnormalities, such as blood dyscrasias, heart defects, hearing loss, and mental retardation. Most doctors recommend vaccination before pregnancy for women not previously exposed to rubella. If pregnancy occurs before vaccination, tell the woman to consult her doctor or nurse-midwife about serial testing for rubella antibody to detect infection.

Minimizing environmental hazards

Exposure to environmental radiation or chemicals, especially in the early weeks of pregnancy, poses a serious threat to fetal well-being. Instruct a woman to avoid X-rays, even dental X-rays, from the moment she suspects or knows that she's pregnant. Explain that high-dose radiation in utero increases the risk of fetal malformation and childhood leukemia and carcinomas. If a woman is accidentally exposed to radiation or chemicals during pregnancy, try to allay her fears and refer her to appropriate resources.

Exploring choices in childbirth

Parents today frequently choose to control the circumstances of their child's birth. For example, they may question the need for the routine administration of analgesics and anesthetics during labor instead of passively accepting it as part of a prescribed childbirth ritual. Or they

HOME CARE

EXERCISING SAFELY DURING PREGNANCY

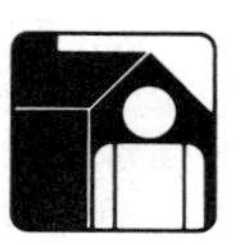

Dear Patient:

Exercising during pregnancy helps you stay healthy and fit. But when you exercise, it's important not to take unnecessary risks that could harm you or your unborn baby. So, to exercise safely during your pregnancy, follow this list of do's and don'ts recommended by the American College of Obstetricians and Gynecologists:

Do:

- Exercise regularly rather than occasionally.
- Perform your exercises on surfaces that reduce shock and provide a sure footing.
- Warm up for 5 minutes before you exercise to stretch your muscles and raise your heart rate gradually. Cool down for 5 minutes, too.
- Measure your heart rate at times of peak activity. It should not exceed 140 beats per minute.
- Drink plenty of fluids before and after you exercise. Interrupt your activity, if necessary, to replenish fluids.
- Begin with mild exercise, if you normally exercise a little or not at all. Then gradually build up to more strenuous exercise.
- Stop any exercise right away and consult your doctor if you develop any of these signs or symptoms: pain, bleeding, dizziness, faintness, shortness of breath, palpitations, or tachycardia (overly rapid heart rate).
- Increase your caloric intake to meet the extra energy demands of pregnancy—and of exercise.
- Plan your exercise program in collaboration with your doctor or nurse-midwife.

Don't:

- Exercise vigorously in hot, humid weather or when you have a fever.
- Perform strenuous exercise for more than 15 minutes.
- Engage in competitive sports.
- Bend deeply or greatly extend your joints.
- Participate in activities that require jumping, bouncing, jarring or jerky motion, or rapid changes in direction.
- Stand up abruptly after doing floor exercises.
- Exercise while lying on your back after the fourth month of pregnancy.
- Perform exercises that use the Valsalva maneuver.
- Exercise beyond your tolerance and comfort level.

may question the choice of a traditional hospital delivery room as the best delivery setting. When you're responsible for preparing a woman for labor and delivery, you'll need to explore childbirth options with her.

However, you'll first teach her how to detect—and correctly respond to—complications of pregnancy or labor and delivery. For example, if the woman is susceptible to toxemia, she should know how to recognize its early signs, such as rapid weight gain, headaches, or ankle or eyelid edema. And she should know to seek immediate medical attention if her membranes rupture early. To help her cope with complications during labor, explain the role of fetal monitoring. Also prepare her for the possibility of cesarean section.

The delivery

Because 20% of women experience some problem during labor (for example, hemorrhage, toxemia, or fetal anoxia), encourage a woman to select a delivery setting that's equipped to handle emergencies as well as provide the childbirth experience she desires. For example, birth centers are becoming increasingly popular. Usually located in the maternity unit of a hospital or operated by a childbirth association, a birth center offers a homelike environment with quick medical intervention available in an emergency.

Once a woman decides where she'd like to deliver, you'll need to help her prepare for the pain of childbirth. Most researchers agree that the less medication a mother receives during labor and delivery, the more responsive and healthy her baby will be. Encourage the woman to attend childbirth classes to learn how to control pain through breathing and relaxation techniques. But assure her that she can request an anesthetic during labor if pain becomes unbearable. Although not totally without risk, local and regional anesthetics are certainly preferable to a general anesthetic.

Providing postpartum instruction

After a woman delivers, your teaching will focus on postpartum nutrition and exercise as well as infant care, such as feeding and safety. For example, remind the mother and her partner to always use an infant car seat, beginning with the baby's trip home from the hospital.

Balancing nutrition and exercise

After delivery, many women think they can immediately resume their pre-pregnancy fitness program and start dieting to lose the weight gained during pregnancy. You'll need to stress the importance of *slowly* resuming exercise to avoid excessive fatigue. If a woman is breast-feeding, she should avoid dieting, which may interfere with her milk production as well as jeopardize her health.

Breast or bottle?

Because breast milk contains a unique balance of nutrients, it's considered the ideal food for infants. What's more, the maternal antibodies it contains help protect the infant against allergy and infection.

When a mother chooses to breast-feed, first explain the physiology of stimulating milk flow. Then teach her how to care for her breasts to prevent soreness and cracked nipples; how to position herself, place the infant at her breast, and stimulate him to suck; and how long to nurse on each breast. Also refer her to a local chapter of a support group, such as Nursing Mothers, for help with problem solving as she adjusts to breast-feeding. If a mother wishes to continue breast-feeding after returning to work, explain how to express breast milk and store it properly. Or, if she wishes to supplement her breast milk or opts not to breast-feed, teach her how to choose and prepare a commercial formula to ensure adequate nutrition. Also teach her the proper technique for bottle-feeding her infant.

Introducing solids

Inform parents that breast milk or formula (with appropriate vitamin and mineral supplements) is the only food their infant needs until he reaches age 3 to 6 months. Explain that introducing solid food too early can cause choking and food allergies and may predispose the infant to obesity.

When the infant's ready for solid food, teach parents to read commercial baby food labels for salt and sugar content. Also instruct them never to add salt or sugar to their infant's food.

To help parents learn what foods their infant likes or dislikes and to determine what foods may cause allergy, teach them to introduce foods in this order: rice cereal, then fruits and vegetables, and finally meats.

Dealing with special problems

Crib death, or sudden infant death syndrome (SIDS), is a chief cause of infant mortality, especially in those from 3 weeks to 7 months old. Typically, parents put the infant to bed and later find him dead, often with no indications of a struggle or distress of any kind. Even an autopsy doesn't reveal the cause of SIDS. Some infants may have had symptoms of a cold or another upper respiratory tract infection, but such symptoms are unusual. Although infants who die from SIDS often appear healthy, research suggests that many may have had undetected abnormalities, such as respiratory immaturity or dysfunction.

When an infant has a history of apneic periods, he's considered at risk for SIDS. You'll need to teach his parents about apnea monitoring. Also instruct them how to perform infant cardiopulmonary resuscitation. (Learning this skill is equally important for all parents. Why? Because suffocation from inhaling food or a small object is another common cause of infant mortality.)

When SIDS claims an infant, you'll need to focus on supporting the grief-stricken parents. Begin by reassuring them that they were not to blame. Provide basic information about SIDS and explain why an autopsy is necessary to confirm the diagnosis. Make sure the parents receive the autopsy report promptly. Then refer them to a local support group for SIDS.

HEALTH IN CHILDHOOD

Perhaps more than any other stage of life, childhood has a profound impact on health. During this period, an individual acquires many habits that may produce lifelong benefit—or harm. To promote healthy habits, you'll need to teach parents how to role-play with their child about significant issues, such as smoking. This open communication can prepare a child to confront the peer-group pressure that so often dominates adolescence.

Developing sound nutritional habits

Usually, a child establishes his eating habits at an early age. Because poor eating habits can affect his growth and development, your teaching must stress the importance of sound nutrition during childhood. You'll also need to explain to parents how poor eating habits contribute to adult disease.

Begin by clearing up any misconceptions about eating habits. For example, tell parents that they shouldn't salt, butter, or sugar their child's food. Although they may prefer their food this way, these acquired tastes increase the child's risk of cardiovascular disease and dental caries.

Because a child needs protein and calcium for growth, parents were once encouraged to supply plenty of eggs, cheese, meat, whole milk, and ice cream in the diet. Research now shows that such a high-cholesterol, high-fat diet increases the risk of atherosclerosis. Therefore, urge parents to serve low-fat alternatives, such as skim milk, lean meat, poultry, and fish. Also suggest that they curb their child's consumption of nonnutritive snacks, such as candy and potato chips.

Teach parents to include a variety of foods in their child's diet to meet his vitamin needs. For example, milk, fish, liver, leafy green vegetables, and yellow fruits and vegetables supply vitamin A. Protein-rich foods, such as meat, and enriched breads and cereals supply the B-complex vitamins. Good sources of vitamin C include citrus fruits, tomatoes, raw cabbage, and green peppers. Fortified milk supplies vitamin D.

To help parents build good eating habits in their child, urge them to follow these tips:

- Serve food portioned out, instead of family style.
- Keep salt off the table.
- Never force a child to eat everything on his plate.
- If a child refuses to eat a certain food, try offering him an alternative from the same food group.
- Keep fresh raw vegetables, such as carrot sticks, ready for snacking.
- Praise a child for his healthy food choices.
- Recognize that a child will imitate his parents' eating habits. So try to avoid using salt, sugar, and butter on your own food, too.

Preventing childhood accidents

Each year, many children die or are injured as the result of automobile and recreational accidents, drownings, fires, and poisoning. Many of these deaths and injuries could have been prevented by

HOME CARE

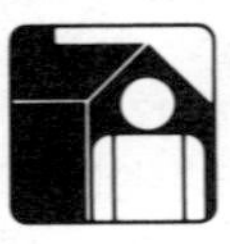

CHILDPROOFING YOUR HOME

Dear Parent:

As a parent, you know how quickly an active toddler can get into trouble. To protect your child, take these simple—but very important—precautions.

How to prevent burns

• Keep matches and lighters out of your child's reach.
• Don't let him play in the kitchen, unless he's in a playpen. You may trip over him or his toys, spilling hot food on him.
• Make sure electrical cords don't hang over counters, tables, or ironing boards. Your child may pull a hot toaster, iron, or Crockpot on himself.
• Don't let pot handles stick out over the edge of the stove. Your child may grab at them.

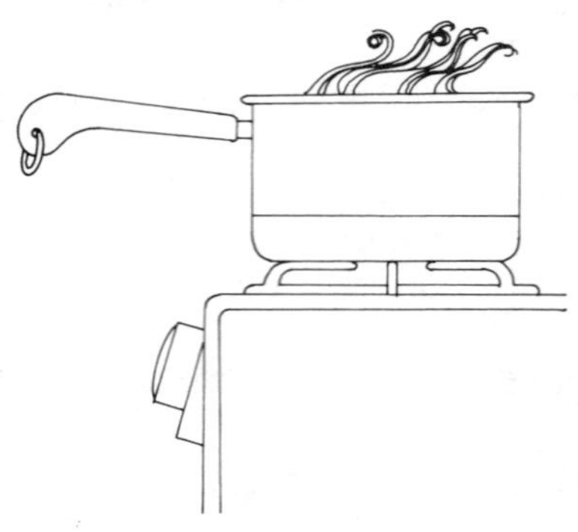

• Don't store candy or cookies on the stove or behind it—your child may try to climb on the stove to find them.
• Don't use tablecloths. A toddler may try to pull himself up by grabbing a tablecloth and pull everything on the table on top of him.

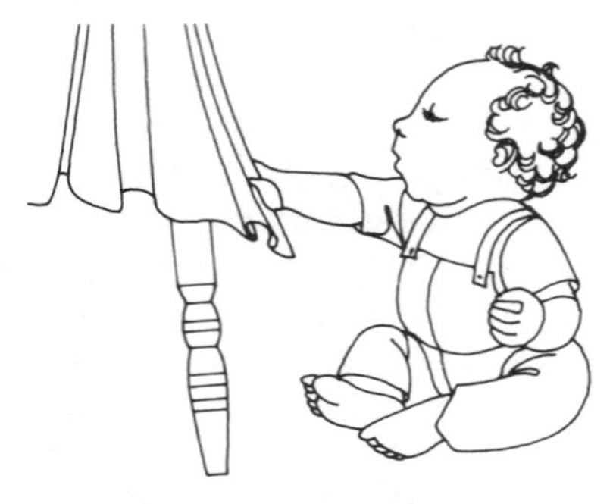

• Don't hold your child while drinking hot coffee or tea—or anything hot. If he bumps your arm, you may splash him with hot liquid.
• Don't leave your child alone in the bathtub—even for an instant. Remember, a child likes to turn knobs. He may turn on the hot-water faucet and burn himself. As an extra precaution, make sure your hot-water heater is set no higher than 130° F. (54.4° C.).
• Check labels on your child's clothing and bedding. Make sure all clothing and bedding are nonflammable.

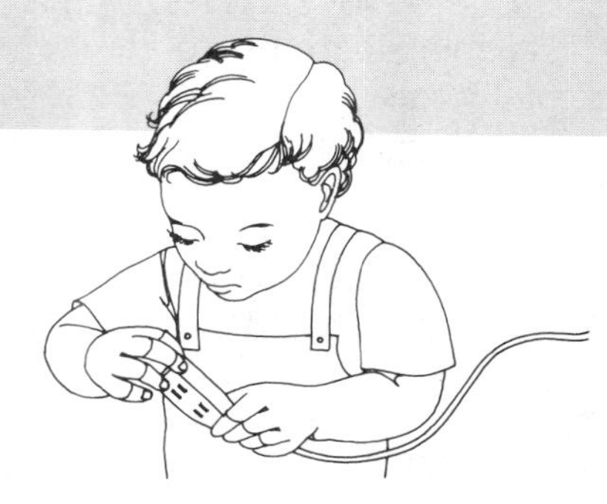

• Don't let him play with—or chew on—electrical cords, including extension cords.
• Be especially careful during holidays. Keep your child away from Christmas tree lights and cords. Don't allow him to play with fireworks or sparklers. And keep him away from flames, including candle flames, when he's dressed in a Halloween costume, especially a homemade costume.

How to prevent poisoning
• Teach your child that everything within reach is not good to eat. To prove the point, give him a taste of something bitter (such as vinegar) on the tip of your finger—but be sure to warn him that it *doesn't* taste good.
• Place poison identification stickers on all household poisons, such as cleaning solutions, polishes, weed spray, and bug killers. Lock them up, or store them on the top shelf of a closet or cabinet—out of reach. (Take care to store them away from food or eating utensils.) After using any poisonous product, *immediately* return it to a safe storage place.

Also keep cosmetics, such as nail polish, perfume, and hand cream, as well as all aerosol containers, out of your child's reach.
• Learn how to identify poisonous plants, and remove any you may find in your home or yard. Remember, many common houseplants, including dieffenbachias, are poisonous when eaten.

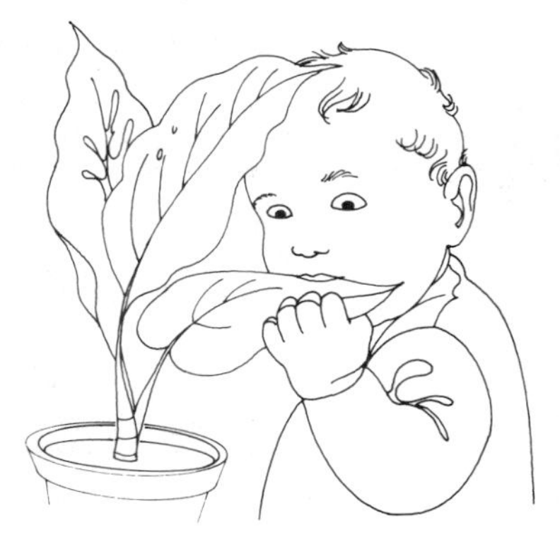

• If your child eats or drinks anything that may be poisonous, immediately call your local poison control center for help. Write the phone number on a label and tape it to the phone. Keep ipecac syrup handy in case the poison control center tells you to make your child vomit what he's swallowed.

observing proper safety measures. For example, a child can be taught how to float and swim or how to safely enjoy bicycles, swings, and other recreational equipment. Teaching parents about such safety measures ranks among your chief goals.

Encourage use of seat belts

More children die in automobile accidents than from any other single cause. That's why you'll need to stress the importance of *consistently* using a car seat for an infant or a young child and a seat belt for an older child. Tell parents that holding a child on their lap doesn't provide enough protection. Even at low driving speeds, the force of impact in a car crash can throw the child through the windshield or into the dashboard. Encourage parents to buckle up as an example for their child to follow.

Refer parents to the state department of transportation for guidance in selecting a car seat. The car seat should be crash-tested and should meet federal safety standards. It must also be suitable for the child's age and size and be installed properly.

SCHEDULE FOR CHILDHOOD IMMUNIZATIONS

Usually, childhood immunizations are given on a fixed schedule, as follows:

AGE	IMMUNIZATION
2 months	First dose: diphtheria/pertussis/tetanus (DPT) vaccine, polio vaccine
4 months	Second dose: DPT vaccine, polio vaccine
6 months	Third dose: DPT vaccine, polio vaccine
15 months	Measles, mumps, and rubella vaccine
18 months	DPT vaccine booster, polio vaccine booster
2 years	*Hemophilus influenzae B* vaccine
4 years	DPT vaccine booster, polio vaccine booster

Before immunization, ask the parent if the child receives corticosteroids or other drugs that depress the immune response, or if he's had a recent febrile illness. Obtain a history of allergies, especially to antibiotics, eggs, or feathers, and past reaction to immunization.

After immunization, tell the parents to watch for and report a severe reaction. Give them a record of their child's immunizations.

Warn against accidental poisoning

Thanks to the advent of lead-free paints and child-proof containers, fewer children die each year from accidental poisoning. However, poisoning still accounts for 5% of accidental deaths in children less than 5 years old. What can you do to improve this statistic? You can begin by teaching parents to place potentially poisonous products, such as household cleaners, bleaches, drugs, and pesticides, well out of the reach of children. Also warn them about lead poisoning, as appropriate. Typically, city children are at an increased risk for lead poisoning because they may ingest chipping lead-base paint from older buildings or inhale lead from automobile exhaust. Explain how lead poisoning damages the central nervous system, possibly leading to learning disabilities, mental retardation, or death. Recommend that parents strip any lead-base paint from walls, molding, and windowsills and then repaint these areas.

Forming good exercise habits

While today's children appear healthy and are taller and heavier than previous generations, they often score poorly on tests of strength, endurance, and agility. Why? Because they're primed at an early age for a sedentary life-style. For example, instead of walking, they're often taxied by their parents to wherever they want to go. What's more, they frequently substitute an afternoon in front of the television for outdoor physical activity.

How can you help parents and children appreciate the benefits of exercise? First, teach them that exercise helps prevent constipation, stress, and obesity. It delays degenerative and cardiovascular disease later in life. And enhances good health by promoting strength, stamina, speed, agility, coordination, and balance.

Then encourage parents to support or initiate an exercise program that suits their child's abilities and interests. To improve cardiovascular fitness, recommend endurance exercises, such as swimming, cycling, running, jumping rope, walking, or hiking. Ideally, the child should choose an exercise that he enjoys and in which he excels. Advise parents against unduly pressuring their child to win when he engages in competitive exercise. Also urge them to make exercise a family activity so that it becomes a healthy habit for the child. Remind them not to rely completely on school physical education programs to promote adequate exercise.

Learning to deal with stress

Even a very young child can experience stress, which may cause depression and jeopardize his psychological well-being. Stress also increases blood pressure and makes a child more susceptible to illness, such as streptococcal infection. To minimize these effects, your teaching must emphasize how to cope with stress effectively and, better yet, how to prevent it.

The most potentially stressful events in a child's life are divorce of his parents and illness or death in his family. Of course, he has no control over these events. However, he can choose to respond to them in either a healthy or a self-destructive way. Teach parents how to communicate with their child and to encourage him to turn to them for help when he's under stress. Also encourage parents to involve their child in school or community activities to help prevent stress.

To enhance a child's psychological well-being, suggest that parents devise projects and games that stimulate curiosity and creativity. Recommend that they limit the child's time for watching television and try to select educational shows. Also encourage parents to spend quality time with their child, especially if both work outside the home. Suggest that they spend the dinner hour with their child and regularly plan family activities.

HEALTH IN ADOLESCENCE

The adolescent years are often trying for both a teenager and his family. As he passes from childhood into adulthood, a teenager develops his own set of values and sense of identity, chiefly by testing and experimenting. Little by little, he withdraws from the family and asserts his independence. Typically, a teenager is motivated by a strong desire to belong to his peer group. He's also overly self-conscious about his appearance—largely a result of sexual maturation during adolescence.

These dramatic changes during adolescence can certainly affect a teenager's health. As a result, you'll need to teach about such varied health problems as poor nutrition, teenage pregnancy, and alcohol and drug abuse.

Meeting growing nutritional demands

Because a teenager's body is growing so rapidly, he needs more calories than he did as a child. However, his diet should still be well balanced and varied. Recommend extra milk to supply needed calcium and protein for growth. When menstruation begins, suggest an iron supplement if adequate iron isn't provided by the diet.

Peer pressure makes food fads common among teenagers. Don't discourage a teenager from following such fads unless they jeopardize his health. Teach him about basic food groups to ensure a balanced diet and healthy weight. Most teenagers don't have a weight problem, but some are obese or suffer from anorexia nervosa.

Obesity

To help an obese teenager, first explore whether his weight problem results from inactivity, overeating, or both. Then try to encourage self-confidence so that he'll be motivated to lose weight. Stress that weight loss is crucial for good health and will also help him feel less ostracized by his peers. Refer him to a local weight-control program.

Anorexia nervosa

Sometimes an obese teenager or one who has a morbid fear of being fat develops a self-starvation disorder known as anorexia nervosa. Most common in teenage girls, this disorder may be life-threatening if untreated. Typically, the affected teenager is preoccupied with food but doesn't allow herself to eat even though she's emaciated. At the same time, she exercises compulsively. She may also demonstrate binge-eating, followed by spontaneous or self-induced vomiting or self-administration of laxatives. Because anorexia is a nutritional problem based on an emotional disturbance, it requires medical and psychiatric treatment. Refer the teenager and her family to Anorexia Nervosa and Associated Disorders (ANAD) for help in treating this disorder.

Preventing teenage suicide

Suicide, the third leading cause of death among teenagers, is usually accomplished by self-inflicted gunshot wounds, drug overdose, or carbon monoxide poisoning by automobile exhaust fumes. Most teenagers who successfully commit suicide have made previous attempts. What's more, a teenager will typically give warning signs of his intentions. Teach parents about such signs and advise them to seek counseling immediately if their teenager demonstrates these signs. Also suggest that parents keep guns and potentially lethal drugs properly secured.

Addressing contraception and teenage pregnancy

Each year about half a million American teenagers give birth, commonly to an infant whose conception wasn't planned. Still other teenagers choose to have an abortion rather than carry an unwanted fetus. To help prevent an unwanted pregnancy, you'll need to provide basic information about how conception occurs and, most important, how it can be avoided.

Methods of contraception

If you're teaching a teenager about contraception, explain that the most effective form of birth control besides abstinence is the oral contraceptive. However, it can produce serious side effects, such as blood clots, CVA, and myocardial infarction (MI). These side effects, though, most commonly occur in women over age 35 or in those who are obese, who smoke more than 15 cigarettes a day, or who have hypertension, diabetes, or elevated serum lipid levels. Outline these risk factors, and encourage yearly gynecologic checkups.

Explain that the next most effective form of birth control is the intrauterine device. Somewhat less effective, but still satisfactory, are the diaphragm, the condom, and spermicides. Inform the teenager that using two of these forms of birth control at the same time improves effectiveness.

WARNING

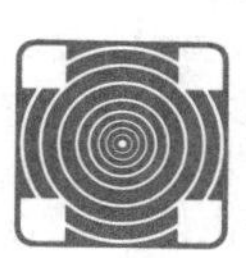

DANGER SIGNS OF TEENAGE SUICIDE

More than likely, you've read or heard about cases in which a teenage boy or girl commits suicide. Sometimes, young lovers or friends even commit suicide together. Do these adolescents leave any warning signs of their intentions? Quite often, they do. You should be aware of these signs—and teach parents how to recognize them. Consider the possibility of a suicide attempt if an adolescent:

- talks frequently about death or about the futility of life
- exhibits dramatic mood changes
- appears sad or downcast, or expresses feelings of hopelessness
- shows loss of interest in his friends or previous activities
- becomes increasingly withdrawn or spends more and more time alone
- begins having trouble at school or receiving poorer grades than usual
- exhibits behavioral changes that suggest alcohol or drug abuse
- starts giving away his prized possessions
- seems unusually apathetic about the future.

Teach parents never to take any behavior for granted. And encourage them to follow their instincts. If they think something is wrong with their son or daughter, they're probably right. They shouldn't try to rationalize or deny any behavior. If they suspect a problem, tell them to seek professional help. Also stress the need to maintain communication with their child.

Teenage pregnancy

Teenage mothers are more likely than adult mothers to have premature or LBW infants and to develop toxemia. The mortality for their infants is also higher. One reason for this trend is that teenage mothers tend to delay seeking prenatal care and thus frequently don't realize the importance of proper nutrition during pregnancy.

You'll need to teach the pregnant teenager how her eating habits affect her unborn child. Explain that she needs extra calories—especially protein and calcium—to sustain her own growth spurts during adolescence as well as promote fetal growth. Emphasize that these calories should be supplied by a well-balanced, nutritious diet.

Curbing the rise of characteristic adolescent problems

Adolescence is a time of exploration and turmoil. Unfortunately, this combination too often leads to behavior that's dangerous to an adolescent and to others.

Motor vehicle accidents

Despite increased public awareness, alcohol-related motor vehicle accidents still rank as the leading cause of teenage deaths. Among other factors that contribute to these deaths are driving under the influence of marijuana or other drugs, driving too fast, and disregarding seat belts. Although driver education programs teach adolescents about safety, you too can promote sensible driving. For example, encourage a teenager to obey the speed limit, to always use a seat belt, and to wear a helmet when riding a motorcycle.

Alcohol and drug abuse

An estimated 3 million American youths between ages 14 and 17 are considered problem drinkers—that is, they become intoxicated at least once a month. Although teenagers drink less often than adults, they tend to drink larger quantities and thus are more apt to become intoxicated when they drink.

Teenagers today consume 30% more alcohol than they did 30 years ago. Not surprisingly, drug abuse is also on the rise. In fact, nearly 30% of youths between ages 12 and 17 have tried marijuana, with 10% of these smoking it every day. Among other substances that teenagers can abuse are amphetamines, cocaine, heroin, hallucinogens, and various illegally obtained prescription drugs.

As a nurse, you must educate both the teenager and his parents about the dangers of alcohol and drug abuse. Encourage parents to help their teenager cope with stress and develop enough self-confidence to say "no" despite peer pressure. When you discover that a teenager is abusing alcohol or drugs, refer him to a local Alcoholics Anonymous chapter, or suggest a rehabilitation center to help him overcome his dependence.

Smoking

Coinciding with the nationwide decline in the number of smokers, fewer teenagers smoke today than in previous years. In fact, smoking is becoming less socially acceptable, as laws passed to prohibit smoking in certain public areas confirm.

Why do some teenagers continue to smoke? Among other reasons, they may smoke to assert their independence, to act grown-up, or to imitate their friends. Also, teenagers are twice as likely to smoke if their parents smoke.

Take every opportunity to teach teenagers and their parents about the dangers of smoking. Explain how smoking shortens life expectancy and increases the risk of cardiovascular disease and lung cancer. When appropriate, refer the teenager to a community program to help him quit smoking.

Encouraging exercise

The benefits of exercise during adolescence are many: it helps the teenager maintain a healthy weight, gives him an outlet for stress, and provides an opportunity to socialize with his peers. Because exercise isn't compatible with smoking and drug and alcohol use, it also tends to discourage him from practicing these unhealthy habits.

Encourage the teenager to take up an exercise—such as tennis or swimming—that he can continue as an adult. Or encourage him to continue a favored exercise that he began as a child. That way, it will more likely become a habit for him. Remind the teenager to increase his caloric intake to meet the extra energy demands of exercise. Also instruct the teenage girl to wear a properly fitting bra during exercise and the teenage boy to wear an athletic supporter.

Preventing accidents in team sports

Many teenagers participate in team sports, either at school or in the community. Although team sports teach important skills—such as working together to achieve a goal and sharing the spotlight—they can also increase the teenager's risk of physical injury and psychological stress.

To reduce the risk of physical injury, urge coaches and community sponsors to invest in and maintain proper equipment, such as helmets, mouthpieces, and shoulder pads. Also emphasize the importance of a clean and safe sports facility. Advise coaches to become certified in first aid so that they can respond promptly to any injury.

Before a teenager participates in a team sport, instruct him to have a complete physical examination. Then stress the importance of proper conditioning to promote better performance and to reduce the risk of injury. For example, to play football, a sport that requires strength, endurance, and agility, a teenager should perform a combination of aerobic and anaerobic exercises, such as running, calisthenics, and weight lifting. Remind him that conditioning also involves proper sleep and nutrition and rules out smoking and alcohol or drug use.

To minimize psychological stress, advise parents not to push a teenager to participate and excel in sports against his will. Teach them to support any interest in sports by encouraging the teenager to practice and to do the best he can. However, they should avoid placing him under stress to perform, to win, or to secure a spot on a specific team.

HEALTH IN ADULTHOOD

Adults in the prime of their lives—between ages 25 and 64—often fall victim to a number of health problems, such as heart disease, CVA, and cancer. Although genetic predisposition contributes to some of these problems, many are linked to specific unhealthy habits, such as overeating, smoking, and lack of exercise. Your teaching can help an adult recognize and correct these habits to help ensure a longer—and healthier—life.

Preventing poor nutrition

Once acquired, poor eating habits are especially difficult to change. To help an adult establish healthy eating habits, teach him to:

- include just enough calories each day to maintain a healthy weight
- limit saturated fats, cholesterol, salt, and sugar in his diet
- eat plenty of complex carbohydrates (whole grains, cereals, fruits, and vegetables)
- substitute more fish, poultry, and legumes (beans, peas, and peanuts) for red meat.

The link between diet and disease

Research shows that a strong correlation exists between diet and certain diseases, such as atherosclerosis, hypertension, and obesity. By teaching an adult how to modify his eating habits, you can help him reduce his risk of acquiring or aggravating such diseases.

- ***Cardiovascular disease.*** Encourage the adult to limit the amount of saturated fats and cholesterol in his diet. Increased serum cholesterol levels are clearly associated with atherosclerosis, which predisposes to MI and CVA. Stress that by modifying his diet an adult can retard, and possibly reverse, atherosclerosis.

To help prevent or control hypertension, instruct the adult to limit salt in his diet. For example, tell him to substitute herbs and other seasonings for salt when cooking and to avoid high-sodium prepared foods.

• ***Cancer.*** Research suggests that a high intake of animal protein or an inadequate intake of fiber may be associated with colon cancer. A high intake of saturated and unsaturated fats also may be linked to colon cancer as well as to ovarian and prostate cancer.

• ***Obesity.*** About 35% of adult women and 13% of adult men are considered obese. Besides being a social stigma, obesity is associated with a number of health problems, such as diabetes, gallbladder disease, and hypertension.

To help the obese adult, you'll need to stress the importance of *permanently* changing his eating habits. Otherwise, he's likely to become trapped in a cycle of losing and then regaining weight. Help him set realistic weight-loss goals and plan a dietary and exercise program to achieve these goals. Also refer him to a community support group, such as Weight Watchers.

Combating inactivity

To promote cardiovascular fitness, an adult should exercise vigorously at least three times a week for 20 to 30 minutes. Unfortunately, most adults get little exercise at work or at home. Your teaching can help an adult understand the many benefits of a regular exercise program. Explain that exercise improves circulation and helps the heart and lungs function more efficiently. By helping the body metabolize carbohydrates and fats, exercise may reduce the risk of atherosclerosis. It can also make an adult feel more energetic, improve his ability to cope with stress, and help him get a good night's sleep. By burning calories and controlling appetite, exercise helps achieve and maintain a healthy body weight and increases muscle strength and stamina.

However, exercise can aggravate hidden or existing health problems and heighten the risk of injuries. So instruct the adult to consult his doctor before starting an exercise program if he:

• has diagnosed heart disease or a heart murmur, or has had an MI

• feels pain or pressure in the chest, left side of the neck, or left shoulder or arm during or after exercise

- feels faint or has dizzy spells
- experiences extreme breathlessness after mild exertion
- is hypertensive or hasn't had his blood pressure checked recently
- has bone or joint problems, such as arthritis
- is a male older than age 45 or a female older than age 50 who isn't used to vigorous exercise
- has a family history of coronary artery disease
- has any other medical condition, such as diabetes.

Refer the adult to the American Heart Association for brochures to teach him how to start an exercise program safely, what exercises he might enjoy, and how to avoid injuries.

Pointing out adult safety risks

In daily living, adults face a number of safety risks, such as toxic environmental agents, occupational hazards, and certain infectious diseases. Accidental injuries can also be potentially life-threatening or disabling. Some safety risks—like toxic waste disposal—are beyond the scope of individual action and require a community effort to affect them. Other risks can be minimized simply by following certain safety measures. For example, teach an adult to use a seat belt consistently, to read product warning labels, and to wear safety goggles when operating machinery. As always, encourage common sense to help prevent accidents. Also teach him precautions against infection, such as hand washing, and urge vaccination when appropriate.

Stress

Occasional stress during adulthood is normal and, in fact, helps an individual respond to his environment and improve his performance. However, chronic or overwhelming stress can tax his ability to cope, resulting in alcohol or drug abuse, depression or mental illness, hypertension, and GI upset.

Research shows that too many stressors occurring at once or consecutively can produce a cumulative effect that increases an individual's chances of becoming ill. Encourage the adult to plan stressors so that they're easier to manage. For example, suggest that a couple delay having a baby if they've just moved into a new home.

- ***Coping skills.*** Teach the adult specific skills to cope with stress, such as cognitive restructuring. This involves focusing on the positive side of events and downplaying the negative. For example, instead of viewing a traffic jam as a hardship and a waste of time, an individual can consider it an opportunity to relax and listen to music.

Point out that distractions, such as humor, reduce stress. Relaxation techniques can help, too. Suggest meditation, or teach the adult how to perform abdominal breathing. If he lives alone, you might recommend getting a pet. Research shows that petting a cat or dog can significantly reduce blood pressure and stress.

However, one of the most important coping skills that you can teach an adult is time management. By managing his time effectively, he can gain a sense of control over his life. Begin by teaching an adult how to set priorities. Tell him to decide what is crucial to him, then to concentrate on that alone. Emphasize that he mustn't feel guilty when he can't accomplish everything. Also advise him to divide unpleasant tasks into small, manageable portions.

Smoking

Since the 1964 Surgeon General's report conclusively linked cigarette smoking to lung cancer, more than 30 million people have quit the habit. However, cigarette smoking remains the largest single cause of preventable illness and premature death. Smokers risk developing heart disease, CVA, chronic lung disease (such as emphysema), and cancer of the lung or other organs. In addition, smokers have a 70% greater chance of premature death than nonsmokers.

To encourage an adult to kick the habit, discuss these health hazards associated with smoking. Also point out the benefits of not smoking; for example, a nonsmoker can enjoy the taste of food more and isn't bothered by tobacco breath odor. Advise the smoker to ask his doctor about the use of nicotine resin complex gum to help him quit smoking. This prescription gum helps the smoker reduce blood levels of nicotine gradually, thereby minimizing withdrawal symptoms. Refer the smoker to the American Cancer Society for more information and support.

Teaching early signs of illness

Part of your responsibility as a nurse is to teach adults about early signs of illness—especially cancer, MI, and CVA. By doing so, you help ensure prompt treatment, which can be lifesaving.

Signs of cancer

Teach the adult about the following types of cancer and their signs.

• ***Breast cancer.*** One out of 11 women develops breast cancer. What's more, it accounts for more cancer deaths in women than any other cancer. So you'll need to emphasize the importance of early detection through monthly breast self-examination and mammography. Explain that mammography can detect small lesions as well as cancer of the regional lymph nodes. The American Cancer Society recommends a baseline mammogram for women between ages 35 and 40. After that, a woman should have a routine mammogram as recommended.

• ***Uterine cancer.*** Thanks to the Pap smear and regular gynecologic checkups, deaths from uterine cancer have decreased by more than 70% over the past 40 years. The American Cancer Society recommends a Pap smear once every 3 years after a woman has had two negative tests performed 1 year apart. Explain that the Pap smear is especially effective in detecting cervical cancer. If a woman's at risk for endometrial cancer, though, her doctor may recommend an endometrial biopsy when she reaches menopause. Also instruct her to watch for warning signs of uterine cancer, such as unusual bleeding or discharge, and to notify her doctor if such signs develop.

• ***Lung cancer.*** Unfortunately, lung cancer is typically well advanced by the time it causes symptoms. As a result, focus your teaching on high-risk groups: smokers, especially if they've had the habit for more than 20 years, and adults exposed to asbestos or other industrial contaminants. Describe the warning signs of lung cancer, including a persistent cough, blood-streaked sputum, and chest pain.

• ***Colorectal cancer.*** Inform the adult that the American Cancer Society recommends these tests for early detection of colorectal cancer: a digital rectal examination performed annually after age 40; a fecal occult blood test performed annually after age 50; and a proctosigmoidoscopy performed every 3 to 5 years after age 50 following two negative annual examinations. Also teach him the warning signs of colorectal cancer: rectal bleeding, bloody stool, or a change in bowel habits.

• ***Testicular cancer.*** This uncommon cancer usually strikes men between ages 20 and 35. To emphasize the importance of monthly testicular self-examination, tell the adult male that 88% of such cancers have already spread by the time they're diagnosed. Also teach him the warning signs of testicular cancer, such as a slight enlargement or a change in the consistency of the testes. A rapidly growing or hemorrhagic cancer may also cause sharp pain or discomfort, often described as "dragging" or "heaviness," in the testes.

• ***Prostate cancer.*** This cancer ranks as the second most common cancer in adult males (lung cancer is first). Describe the warning signs of prostate cancer, such as weak or interrupted urine flow, an inability to urinate or control urine flow, frequency (especially at night), blood-tinged urine, pain or burning on urination, and pain

INQUIRY

QUESTIONS PATIENTS ASK ABOUT P.M.S.

Why do I always feel this way before my menstrual period?

Although doctors aren't sure about the exact cause of premenstrual syndrome (PMS), they think it probably results from hormonal changes—chiefly involving progesterone and estrogen—during the menstrual cycle. Another hormone called prolactin may also contribute to PMS.

Do many other women also experience PMS?

Yes. In fact, up to 70% of women experience PMS. However, it affects each woman differently. Some women have only mild discomfort, while others have severe symptoms. For example, a woman may experience anxiety or panic attacks, depression, irritability, fatigue, food cravings, breast tenderness and swelling, bloating, swollen ankles or fingers, joint aches and pains, headaches, or even seizures.

How can I obtain relief from PMS?

Although your doctor may prescribe certain drugs or exercise to treat symptoms of PMS, you can help, too, by simply watching what you eat. Most important, you should try to steer clear of salt, caffeine, and sugar.

By reducing salt in your diet for 7 to 9 days before your period, you can help reduce water retention associated with uncomfortable bloating. This may also help to ease some of the aches and pains caused by water-swollen tissues pressing against nearby nerves.

Why reduce caffeine in your diet? Because caffeine can worsen the nervousness, irritability, and insomnia that you may already experience with PMS.

Hormonal changes in PMS also seem to affect your body's production of insulin, the hormone that causes your blood sugar level to drop. That's why most doctors recommend that you eliminate all sugars from your diet, including honey, molasses, brown sugar, candy, sweet desserts and snacks, and regular soft drinks. Your doctor may also suggest that you divide your daily caloric intake into three small meals and three between-meal snacks to avoid sudden drops in your blood sugar level.

One more point about what you eat. Because alcohol stimulates the release of insulin, it also can cause your blood sugar level to drop. So most doctors recommend that you avoid alcohol for two weeks before your period. But, if you're going to indulge, remember that you'll need only half your usual amount of alcohol to obtain the same effect. That's because PMS apparently makes you more susceptible to intoxication.

HOME CARE

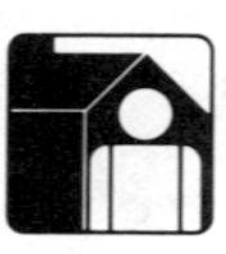

HOW TO EXAMINE YOUR BREASTS

Dear Patient:

Since 90% of breast cancers are discovered by patients themselves, it's important to learn and practice self-examination. You should examine your breasts once a month. If you've not yet reached menopause, the best time is immediately after your menstrual period. If you're past menopause, choose any convenient day.

Here's how to examine your breasts:

1

Undress to the waist, and stand or sit in front of a mirror, with your arms at your sides. Observe your breasts for any change in their shape or size and any puckering or dimpling of the skin.

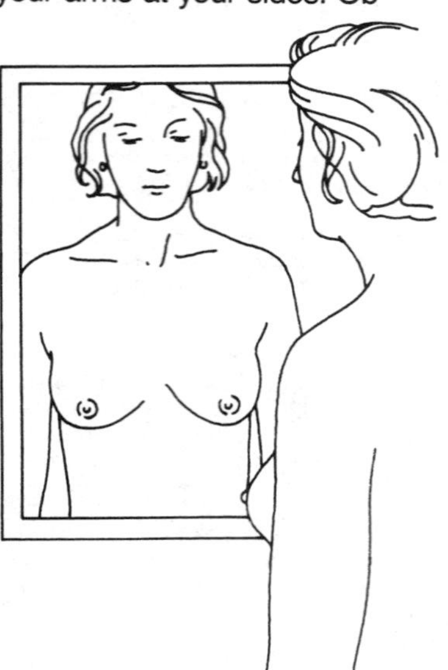

2

Raise your arms and press your hands together behind your head. Observe your breasts as you did before.

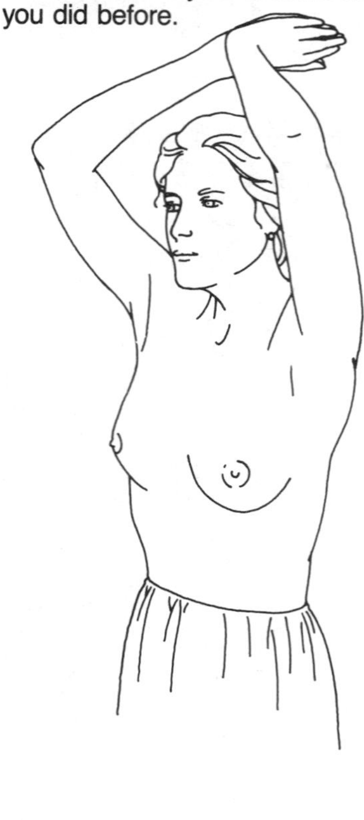

3

Press your palms firmly on your hips and observe your breasts again.

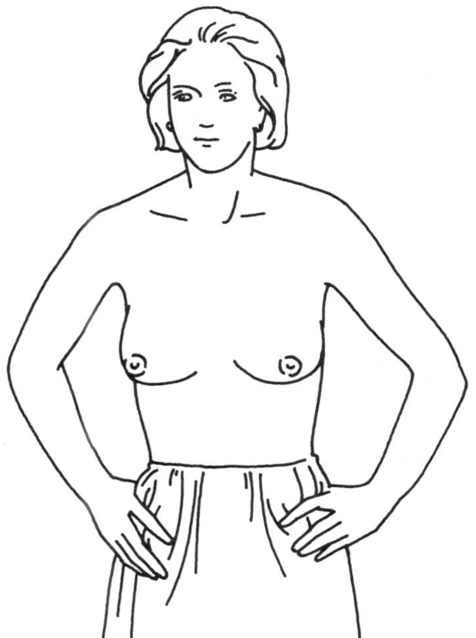

4

Now, lie flat on your back. This position flattens and spreads your breasts more evenly over the chest wall. Place a small pillow under your left shoulder, and put your left hand behind your head.

5

Examine your left breast with your right hand, using a circular motion and progressing clockwise, until you've examined every portion. You'll notice a

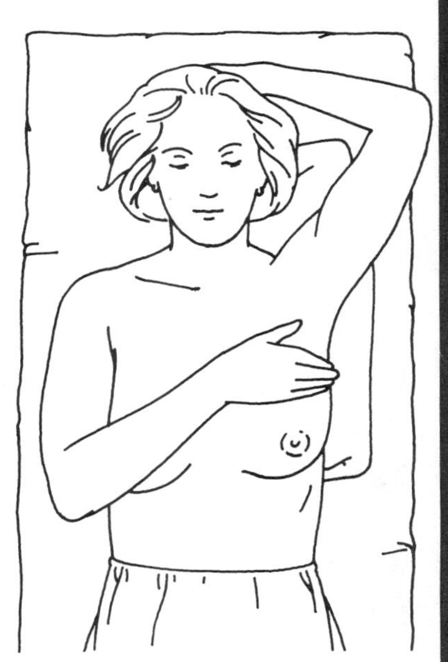

ridge of firm tissue in the lower curve of your breast; this is normal.

(continued)

HOME CARE

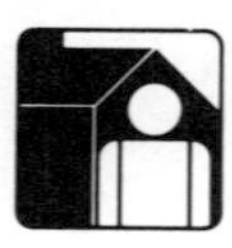

HOW TO EXAMINE YOUR BREASTS *(continued)*

6

Check the area under your arm with your elbow slightly bent.

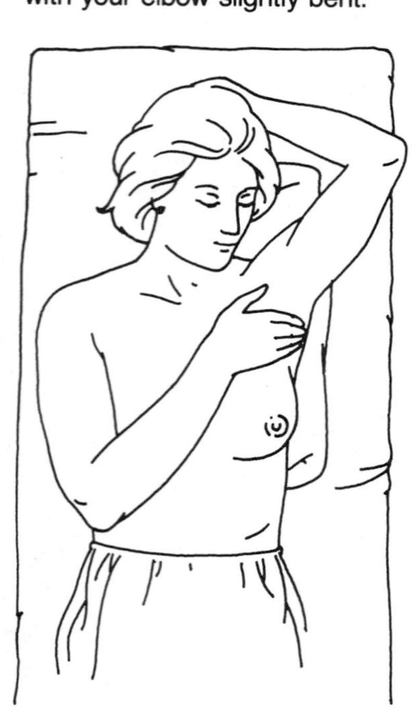

If you feel a small lump under your armpit that moves freely, don't be alarmed. This area contains your lymph glands, which may become swollen when you're sick. Check the size of the lump daily. Call the doctor if it doesn't go away in a few days or if it gets larger.

7

Gently squeeze your nipple between your thumb and forefinger, and note any discharge.

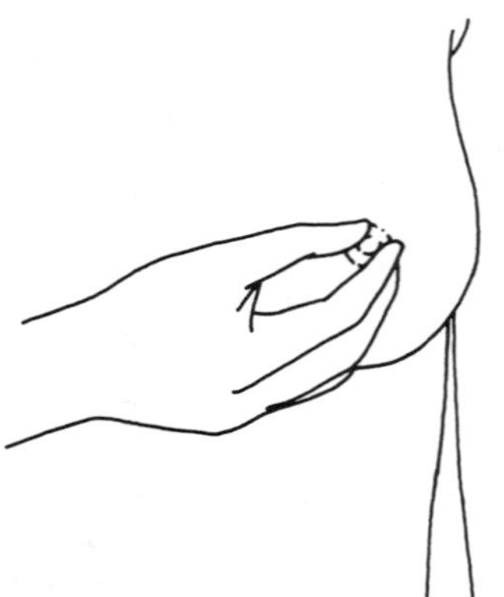

Repeat this examination on your right breast, using your left hand.

8

Finally, examine your breasts while in the shower or bath, lubricating your breasts with soap and water. Using the

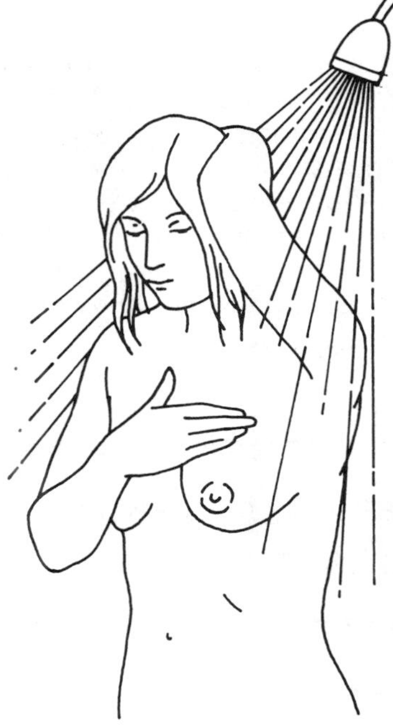

same circular, clockwise motion, gently inspect both breasts with your fingertips. After you've toweled dry, squeeze each nipple gently, and note any discharge.

9

If you feel a lump while examining your breasts, don't panic—most lumps aren't cancerous. First, note whether you can easily lift the skin covering it and whether the lump moves when you do so.

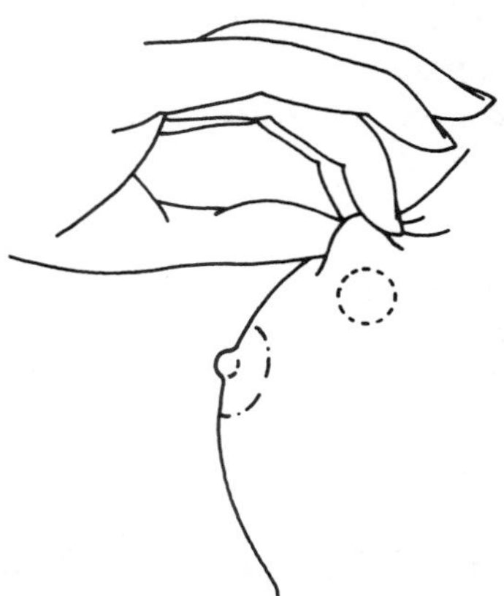

Next, notify your doctor. Be prepared to describe how the lump feels (hard or soft) and whether it moves easily under the skin.

Chances are, your doctor will want to examine the lump. Then he can advise you about what treatment (if any) you need.

Remember, although self-examination is important, it's not a substitute for examination by your doctor. Be sure to see your doctor annually or semiannually (if you're considered at special risk).

in the lower back, pelvis, or upper thighs. If the adult develops any of these signs or symptoms, instruct him to see his doctor to rule out other prostate problems.

Signs of MI

Teach the adult to seek medical help immediately if he experiences MI's cardinal symptom: persistent chest pain (often described as "heavy," "squeezing," or "crushing") that may radiate to the left side of the jaw or neck or to the left shoulder or arm. Mention that MI may also cause anxiety or a sense of impending doom, dizziness or fainting, sweating, nausea, and shortness of breath.

Signs of CVA

Describe these signs of CVA to the adult: sudden, temporary weakness or numbness of the face, arm, or leg on one side of the body; temporary loss of speech or inability to understand speech; temporary loss of vision or blurred vision, usually in one eye; unexplained dizziness, unsteadiness, or sudden falls. Explain that many severe CVAs are preceded by transient ischemic attacks. These attacks produce signs similar to a CVA and may occur days, weeks, or even months before a CVA. If the adult experiences any of these signs, have him notify his doctor promptly to help prevent death or severe disability.

Preventing the spread of sexually transmitted disease

Each year, sexually transmitted disease (STD) strikes 10 million adults, most of them between ages 15 and 30. Although gonorrhea and syphilis are the best known types of STD, genital herpes and nonspecific urethritis (often caused by *Chlamydia*) also infect many adults. Because STD is often asymptomatic, it's difficult to detect and control. Unfortunately, thousands of infected women of childbearing age develop secondary pelvic inflammatory disease, which can cause sterility.

To help prevent and control STD, teach the adult that each type of STD is caused by a different organism. Note that he can have more than one STD at any given time. Remind him that reinfection is possible, too. Explain that condoms and some contraceptive creams and foams may protect against STD. Recommend limiting

HOME CARE

HOW TO EXAMINE YOUR TESTICLES

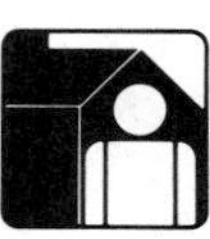

Dear Patient:

To help you detect abnormalities early, you should examine your testicles once a month. Eventually, you'll become familiar with them and will be able to recognize anything abnormal. Here's how to examine your testicles:

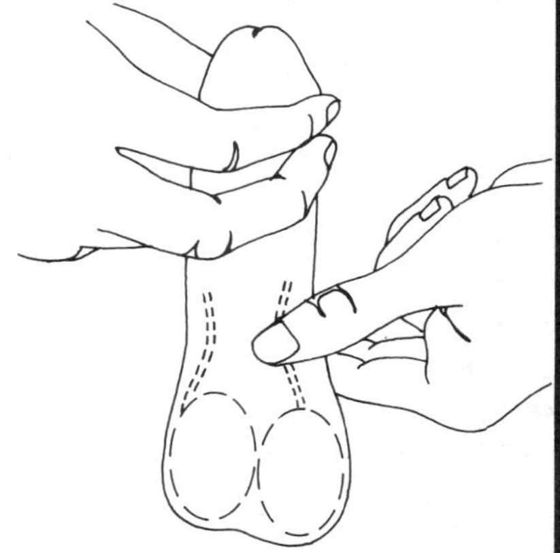

1

Remove your clothes and stand in front of a mirror. With one hand, lift your penis and check your scrotum (the sac containing your testicles) for any change in shape or size and for red, distended veins. Expect the scrotum's left side to hang slightly lower than the right.

2

Next, feel your testicles for lumps and masses. First, locate the cordlike structure at the back of your testicles. This is called the epididymis. Your spermatic cord extends upward from the epididymis.

3

Gently squeeze the spermatic cord above your right testicle between the thumb and first two fingers of your right hand. Then, using the thumb and first two fingers of your left hand, examine the spermatic cord above your left testicle. Check for lumps and masses by squeezing along the entire length of the cords.

4

To examine your right testicle, place your right thumb on the front of the testicle and your index and middle fingers behind it. Gently press your thumb and fingers together; they should meet. Make sure you check your entire testicle. Then, use your left hand to examine your left testicle in the same manner. Your testicles should feel smooth, rubbery, and slightly tender, and you should be able to move them.

If you notice any lumps, masses, or changes, notify your doctor.

sexual contacts, avoiding infected partners, and urinating and cleansing the genitals right after intercourse. Urge an infected adult to inform sexual partners so they can seek treatment.

HEALTH IN OLD AGE

Today, more people live to old age than ever before. Fortunately, only 5% of the elderly need to be institutionalized; the rest can maintain their independence. However, 80% of the elderly suffer from at least one chronic health problem. Your teaching can help them cope with existing health problems as well as avoid new ones. What's more, it can improve their quality of life and help them continue as contributing members of society.

Emphasize that aging is a state of mind as well as of body. Urge the elderly person to continue as many activities as possible, depending on his mobility. Also help him explore new interests or hobbies. Recommend that he attend a hospital- or community-sponsored seminar on retirement. Such seminars usually cover topics like budgeting and health and fitness.

Perhaps the most powerful influence in old age is death. Besides contemplating his own mortality, an elderly person must often face the death of close friends or, most stressful of all, a spouse. By teaching him how to deal with grief, you can help the elderly person come to terms with such losses.

Ensuring proper nutrition

You'll need to suggest ways to help the elderly maintain good nutrition.

Caloric intake

Because metabolism slows with age, an elderly person requires fewer calories than before. However, metabolism still varies widely, so you'll need to help him adjust his caloric intake appropriately. For

HOME CARE

HOW TO SELECT—AND ENJOY—HEALTHFUL FOODS

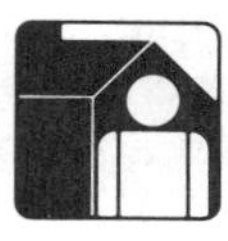

Dear Patient:

A healthful diet means selecting the right foods to meet your body's needs. Here's how:

Selecting the right foods

Rely on the four basic food groups to ensure a healthful diet. The *fruit-vegetable* group includes all fruits and vegetables; the *bread-cereal* group, all grains and everything made from them, such as flour and pasta. The *meat* group includes beef and other meats, fish, poultry, and eggs; the *milk* group, milk and everything made from it, such as cheese, ice cream, and yogurt.

Each day, try to follow the 4-4-2-2 rule: 4 servings from the fruit-vegetable group, 4 servings from the bread-cereal group, 2 servings from the meat group, and 2 servings from the milk group.

Also remember these tips:

- To prevent or relieve constipation, make sure you're getting adequate fiber in your diet. That means eating a variety of fruits and vegetables as well as whole grain bread and foods like brown rice and barley.
- Watch your intake of cholesterol and saturated fats to lower your risk of heart disease. Eat more chicken and turkey (remove the skin), rabbit, and fish rather than beef. And substitute low-fat or skimmed milk, cheeses like cottage cheese and ricotta, and yogurt for whole milk and its products. Just be sure not to neglect the milk group. Why? Because it provides calcium to help prevent your bones from becoming brittle.

Making mealtime more enjoyable

Once you've selected the right foods, follow these tips to make mealtime enjoyable:

- Since your taste buds become less sensitive as you grow older, you may need more seasonings to bring out the flavor in food. Try a variety of seasonings and herbs until you find what you like. However, avoid excessive use of salt, which can cause fluid retention and increase your risk of high blood pressure.
- If you live alone, try to eat with a friend. It's always more enjoyable to prepare a "sit-down" meal for two. You might even plan a picnic if the weather's nice.
- Buy a cookbook or take one out from the library, and plan some easy new meals.

example, if he's moderately active, recommend 5% fewer calories for each decade between ages 40 and 59, 10% fewer calories between ages 60 and 69, and another 10% fewer after age 70.

Fiber and fluids

Encourage the elderly person to include adequate fiber in his diet. Fiber helps prevent constipation—a problem that the elderly are especially prone to because of reduced activity. It may also help prevent colon cancer, diverticulosis, and gallstones.

Because aging decreases the number of functional nephrons, instruct the elderly person to drink adequate fluids to promote excretion. Generally, he should drink 1 ml of water per calorie daily. Explain that he'll need to increase this amount if he's losing more water than usual, for example, with diarrhea, polyuria, use of diuretics, or excessive perspiration.

Vitamins and minerals

Because an elderly person requires fewer calories, he must be especially careful to eat healthful foods to get the vitamins and minerals he needs. Explain that calcium absorption decreases with age, increasing the risk for osteoporosis. To help prevent or delay osteoporosis, encourage the elderly person to increase his calcium intake, as recommended by his doctor. But instruct him not to take a calcium supplement without his doctor's approval.

Conveying the benefits of exercise

Encourage the elderly person to exercise for enjoyment and relaxation as well as to promote cardiovascular health. Explain how exercise can make him feel more energetic, help him cope with stress, and promote a good night's sleep. It also helps keep his joints limber and prevent backache.

Exercises most frequently recommended for the elderly include walking, swimming, bicycling, hiking, jogging, and yoga. When possible, suggest that he ask a friend to join him to make exercise more enjoyable.

Advise the elderly person to see his doctor before starting any exercise program. By performing an exercise stress test, the doctor can evaluate how well the person's heart responds to exercise. Then, to promote safe exercise, encourage him to:

- begin his exercise program gradually over a period of weeks
- never exceed his tolerance level during exercise
- limber up gently and slowly
- be alert for muscle and joint pains as well as early warning signs of MI
- exercise on surfaces that reduce shock and provide a sure footing
- wear well-fitting support shoes
- drink plenty of fluids to replenish water lost through perspiration
- avoid vigorous exercise in hot, humid weather.

Coping with the effects of aging

Many elderly suffer from at least one chronic health problem—most commonly, arthritis, heart or respiratory disease, or impaired vision or hearing. Unfortunately, such problems often occur simultaneously in the elderly, taxing the individual's and his family's ability to cope. Your teaching can encourage an elderly person to perform self-care, when possible, and thereby maintain his independence. It can also guide his family in reallocating chores when disability forces the elderly person to relinquish his former role.

Minimizing the effects of immobility

If an elderly person has limited mobility, do all you can to link him with community services to avoid unnecessary institutionalization. For example, tell him about Meals On Wheels; transportation services to and from the doctor's office, church, or grocery store; homemaker services; and the role of visiting nurses and home health aides.

To help minimize immobility, stress the importance of exercise and a positive attitude. Also teach precautions against falls. For example, urge the elderly person to anchor throw rugs to the floor or to obtain throw rugs that have nonskid backing. Suggest installing grab rails in the bathtub to make getting in and out of the tub much easier—and safer. Applying nonslip strips or decals to the bottom of the tub also helps ensure good footing. Remember, the elderly are prone to fractures when they fall, and their healing time is also delayed.

Compensating for sensory loss

Aging commonly affects an individual's sense of taste, smell, hearing, and sight. That's why you'll need to teach the elderly person how to protect each of these senses and compensate for impaired function.

• ***Taste and smell.*** Research shows that taste buds diminish in number and sensitivity with age. Many elderly also have difficulty distinguishing odors. Because taste and smell contribute so much to food appreciation, an elderly person may develop poor eating habits. To stimulate his appetite, suggest how to arrange food attractively, and encourage him to vary his diet. If an elderly person has dentures, instruct him to see his doctor if he experiences pain when chewing; his dentures may need to be refitted.

• ***Hearing.*** Hearing loss is a widespread problem among the elderly. Unfortunately, they sometimes fall victim to fraud when buying hearing aids without guidance from trained medical personnel. If an elderly person suspects hearing loss, stress the importance of consulting an otolaryngologist or audiologist to determine its cause and proper treatment.

• ***Sight.*** To help an elderly person preserve his sight, stress the importance of routine eye checkups to detect glaucoma and to update his eyeglass prescription. Explain how a current prescription prevents eyestrain during reading and, even more important, promotes safety if he's driving. Encourage him to take advantage of free eye screening at a local health fair. Or suggest that he ask his family for eyeglasses as a Christmas or birthday present.

Preventing infection

Influenza and pneumonia are leading causes of death among the elderly, especially those weakened by chronic health problems. Just consider these statistics: pneumococcal pneumonia is responsible for more than 50,000 deaths a year. Compared to the rest of the population, the death rate is 2½ times higher for those between ages 65 and 74 and 10 times higher for those between ages 75 and 84.

Advise the elderly person to consult his doctor about vaccination against influenza and pneumococcal pneumonia, especially if he has chronic lung disease. Explain that chronic lung disease makes him less able to tolerate respiratory infection. Also remind him of other measures to prevent infection, such as hand washing.

A FINAL WORD

Whether you're addressing an elderly person or a young child, your health teaching can accomplish only so much. After all, it's up to the individual to modify his health habits. You can't force him to stop smoking or to use a seat belt consistently. But you can promote self-responsibility—the key to his willingness to follow your health teaching. To promote self-responsibility, recognize the individual's strengths, and praise his choice of healthy habits. Accept setbacks (for example, when he goes off his diet) without harsh criticism to avoid discouraging him.

Above all, be an example for him to follow by eliminating unhealthy habits from your own life.

SELECTED REFERENCES

Advice for the Patient, 8th ed. Rockville, Md.: United States Pharmacopeial Convention, Inc., 1988.

Drug Information for the Health Care Provider, 8th ed. Rockville, Md.: United States Pharmacopeial Convention, Inc., 1988.

Falvo, D.R. *Effective Patient Education: A Guide to Increased Compliance.* Rockville, Md.: Aspen Systems Corp., 1984.

McCorkle, R., and Germino, N. "What Nurses Need to Know about Home Care," *Oncology Nursing Forum* 11(6):63-69, November/December 1984.

Medication Teaching Manual: A Guide for Patient Counseling, 3rd ed. Bethesda, Md.: American Society of Hospital Pharmacists, 1983.

Rankin, S.H., and Duffy, K., eds. *Patient Education: Issues, Principles, and Guidelines.* Philadelphia: J.B. Lippincott Co., 1983.

Redman, B.K. *The Process of Patient Teaching in Nursing,* 5th ed. St. Louis: C.V. Mosby Co., 1983.

Ruzicki, D.A. "Evaluation: It's What You Do With What You've Got that Counts," *Promoting Health* 6(5):6-9, September/October 1985.

Veenker, C.H. "Evaluating Health Practice and Understanding," *Health Education* 16(2):80-82, February 1985.

Woldum, K., et al. *Patient Education: Foundations of Practice.* Rockville, Md.: Aspen Systems Corp., 1984.

INDEX

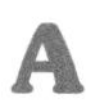

D

i refers to illustration, t refers to table.

i refers to illustration, t refers to table.

J - L

M

N

O

P

i refers to illustration, t refers to table.

Q - R

S

T

U - Z

i refers to illustration, t refers to table.